Pediatric
Telephone Medicine

Second Edition

Pediatric Telephone Medicine

Principles, Triage, and Advice

Jeffrey L. Brown, M.D.

Clinical Associate Professor of Pediatrics
Departments of Pediatrics and Psychiatry
The New York Hospital-Cornell Medical Center
New York, New York

Attending Pediatrician and Past Chairman
Department of Pediatrics
United Hospital Medical Center
Port Chester, New York

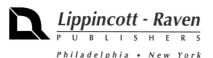

Lippincott - Raven
P U B L I S H E R S

Philadelphia • New York

General
Principles

Common
Symptoms

Emergencies
and Traumas

Minor
Infections

Infectious
Diseases

Parenting
Concerns

Infant
Care

General Principles

Common Symptoms

Emergencies and Traumas

Minor Infections

Infectious Diseases

Parenting Concerns

Infant Care

Acquisitions Editor: Richard Winters
Sponsoring Editor: Jody Schott
Production Editor: Mary Kinsella
Indexer: David Prout
Production Manager: Janet Greenwood
Production Service: Caslon, Inc.
Compositor: The Composing Room of Michigan, Inc.
Printer/Binder: RR Donnelley & Sons, Crawfordsville

Second Edition

Printed in the United States of America

6 5 4 3

Library of Congress Cataloging-in-Publication Data
Brown, Jeffrey L.
  Pediatric telephone medicine: principles, triage, and advice /
Jeffrey L. Brown. — 2nd ed.
      p.   cm.
  Includes bibliographical references and index.
  ISBN 0-397-51379-8
    1. Children—Diseases—Treatment.   2. Telephone in medicine.
I. Title.
    [DNLM: 1. Pediatrics.   2. Child care.   3. Emergencies—in infancy
& childhood.   4. Telephone.   5. Triage.   WS 200 B878p 1994]
RJ370.B76   1994
a618.92—dc20
DNLM/DLC
for Library of Congress   94-15488
                                                                              CIP

Care has been taken to confirm the accuracy of the information presented and to describe generally accepted practices. However, the authors, editors, and publisher are not responsible for errors or omissions or for any consequences from application of the information in this book and make no warranty, express or implied, with respect to the contents of this publication.

The authors, editors, and publisher have exerted every effort to ensure that drug selection and dosage set forth in this text are in accordance with current recommendations and practice at the time of publication. However, in view of ongoing research, changes in government regulations, and the constant flow of information relating to drug therapy and drug reactions, the reader is urged to check the package insert for each drug for any change in indications and dosage and for added warnings and precautions. This is particularly important when the recommended agent is a new or infrequently employed drug.

Some drugs and medical devices presented in this publication have Food and Drug Administration (FDA) clearance for limited use in restricted research settings. It is the responsibility of the health care provider to ascertain the FDA status of each drug or device planned for use in their clinical practice.

Dedicated with love, respect, and gratitude to
Edna and Joel Brown

General
Principles

Common
Symptoms

Emergencies
and Traumas

Minor
Infections

Infectious
Diseases

Parenting
Concerns

Infant
Care

Preface

When the predecessor of this manual was published more than a decade ago, telephone triage and advice had received only minimal attention by professionals and the public. Today, more than half of the accredited pediatric residency programs have some type of training in the triage and management of telephone calls, the American Academy of Pediatrics includes a section on telephone medicine in its manual on *Management of Pediatric Practice,* peer-reviewed articles appear regularly in the professional literature, and a choice of pediatric telephone triage books has become available to practitioners (see the bibliography). In addition, large numbers of parents have come to realize that they rely on the telephone for advice on child rearing and illness. To help them improve their effectiveness at telephone usage, this topic is now addressed regularly on parenting television shows and in parenting books, videotapes, and magazines (see Brown JL: *The Complete Parents' Guide to Telephone Medicine: When To Call, What To Ask, How To Help.* Revised Second Edition. New York: Perigee, 1988).

The first edition of this manual attempted to correct many of the deficiencies of the earlier book. But, after reviewing the growing literature on telephone medicine, rendering expert opinion for many malpractice actions brought against pediatricians, and responding to parents' concerns in an office-based pediatric practice for more than 20 years, we have become convinced that it is necessary to redirect the focus of telephone medicine from the mastering of algorithmic protocols toward equally important skills needed by pediatric practitioners: improving general communication skills, clinical instinct, and patient relations. The net result will be a more friendly and efficient work environment that will also reduce professional liability.

For these reasons, this Revised Second Edition has added new sections that address these topics and expanded others that relate to the practical management of telephone calls. The language used purposefully avoids overly technical terminology so that it can be understood by most ancillary staff likely to respond to parents' telephone calls. And, of course, medical topics have been updated to reflect current thinking about treating common symptoms such as fever and diarrhea.

Pediatricians have taken the lead by emphasizing the important role

General
Principles

Common
Symptoms

Emergencies
and Traumas

Minor
Infections

Infectious
Diseases

Parenting
Concerns

Infant
Care

that the telephone plays in medical practice. We hope that other special-
ties will follow our lead in converting this important clinical skill from
one that had been relegated to "on the job" training to one that shares
equal importance with learning inperson history taking and other aspects
of patient management.

Contents

Common
Symptoms

Emergencies
and Traumas

Minor
Infections

Infectious
Diseases

Parenting
Concerns

Infant
Care

Common Symptoms

Emergencies and Traumas

Minor Infections

Infectious Diseases

Parenting Concerns

Infant Care

General
Principles

Common
Symptoms

Emergencies
and Traumas

Minor
Infections

Infectious
Diseases

Parenting
Concerns

Infant
Care

Pediatric Telephone Medicine

General Principles of Telephone Medicine

Common
Symptoms

Emergencies
and Traumas

Minor
Infections

Infectious
Diseases

Parenting
Concerns

Infant
Care

1

Introduction

The telephone has become an integral part of modern pediatric practice. Parents rely on the telephone to make rapid contact with the doctor, and practitioners orient their professional activities around telephone accessibility. Inefficient telephone use quickly leads to great discontent for both practitioners and patients, and poor telephone management can be the downfall of an otherwise successful practice. A concise, exacting telephone style can be money-saving for parents who will avoid unnecessary office visits and receive better advice; practitioners benefit when fewer patients are seen after-hours, when patient flow improves, and when there is a decreased likelihood of missed diagnosis with resulting liability. Unfortunately, surveys show that even staff from hospital emergency rooms that participate in formal pediatric residency training programs frequently provide inaccurate and haphazard telephoned advice when parents call with potentially serious medical problems.

This manual provides a planned approach for using the telephone as a medical tool and may be especially helpful for group practices and other treatment settings where a relatively uniform response to patient queries is needed. Although patient populations and types of practices vary greatly, the general principles discussed are applicable to most clinical settings. Before use, this or any other telephone triage manual should be carefully reviewed by the physician in charge so that modifications can be made to conform with the practice preferences at that treatment location.

Importance of the Telephone

At a time when more than half of the mothers of preschool-aged children are working outside the home and greater mobility has limited geographic access to relatives, the child's physician has assumed greater importance to parents than ever before. Almost unnoticed, the telephone has become an essential link to successful parenting when constant communication between the workplace, the child's daytime caretaker, and the doctor's office must be maintained.

Jeffrey L. Brown: *Pediatric Telephone Medicine: Principles, Triage, and Advice,* Second Edition. Copyright © 1994 J. B. Lippincott Company

General
Principles

Common
Symptoms

Emergencies
and Traumas

Minor
Infections

Infectious
Diseases

Parenting
Concerns

Infant
Care

Objectives of Telephoned Contacts with Patients

As with other aspects of pediatric practice, it is difficult to develop a strategy for solving the problems associated with telephoned patient contacts unless goals are clearly defined. *Initial primary objectives* should include the maintenance of a high quality of response, the avoidance of missed pathology, the establishment of good patient relations, and the ability to complete a large volume of calls in the shortest period of time. *Other goals* include providing advice that can relieve a child's discomfort, calming distraught parents, reassuring oneself about a child's illness, and encouraging parents to conform to guidelines established by the practice. Parents of hospitalized patients can benefit from frequent telephoned contact with the child's doctor because of his or her increased availability, and parents of children seen as in- and outpatients will appreciate those times when telephoned follow-up can substitute for a follow-up examination. Both office staff and parents benefit when there is improved telephone management of administrative functions that include scheduling appointments, providing basic advice, and maintaining liaison with insurance companies, suppliers, and pharmacies.

Basic Elements of the Telephone Call

It is a common mistake to believe that effective telephoned patient contact only requires mastering a list of screening questions to rule out serious illness. Although screening questions are important, they are only one element among many that should be learned to avoid some very serious telephone management traps. Each call should be thought of as having an *introduction,* a fact-finding and advice-giving *middle,* and a summarizing *conclusion.* Each component is as important as the other and will be considered separately.

The Introduction

The introduction to a telephoned patient contact sets the tone for the rest of the call. A clinician can increase a parent's receptivity to in-person meetings by utilizing appropriate body language, proper dress, and grooming and by placing herself at eye level, *i.e.,* standing when the parent is standing and sitting when the parent is seated. Voice and manner must accomplish the same goals during telephone contacts. The introduction includes a greeting, information gathering, and questions to make a global assessment of the caller and to determine the reason for the call.

Identification
Staff should be instructed to state their own names as well as that of the institution or practice to personalize the message and increase individual accountability. Identification should be coupled with an offer to be of service: "County Pediatric Group. Sally speaking. How can I help you?"

The Greeting
The greeting should be warm and polite. A terse beginning to the call decreases your ability to gather accurate information or convince a parent to follow your advice. "Hi. This is Dr. Smith. How can I help you?" is much more effective than "Dr. Smith here."

The "Hold" Button
Parents should be placed on hold as infrequently and for the shortest period of time possible. Be as respectful of the parent's time as you want

General
Principles

Common
Symptoms

Emergencies
and Traumas

Minor
Infections

Infectious
Diseases

Parenting
Concerns

Infant
Care

them to be of yours. When picking up these calls, an apology is always appreciated: "I'm sorry to keep you waiting. How can I help you?"

Gathering Information

Background information should include the patient's name, age, and sex, the chief complaint or reason for the call, and, when pertinent, chronic illnesses and medicines that are currently being given. In addition, an attempt should be made to make a *global assessment* of the parent's reliability, present state of mind, and level of anxiety. Lastly, the *time of day* should be noted since it may influence the advice given, such as the need to use hospital rather than office services.

The Middle Call

Diagnosis and Triage

Making an accurate *diagnosis* can be helpful but is not nearly as important as making an appropriate disposition to the call. Effective *triage* is one of the most difficult telephone skills to master. As with other clinical skills, it requires a well-coordinated balance of good history taking and clinical knowledge, together with a healthy sprinkling of intuition.

The possible damage caused by delayed treatment of a serious illness is obvious. Much less apparent is the morbidity caused when a parent is instructed to bring his or her child in for an "unnecessary" examination. Overscreening of symptoms can become very expensive when the costs of time away from work, transportation, baby-sitting, and other arrangements are added to the dollar amount of the visit. Unfortunately, lack of clinician reimbursement for telephone time may become a factor in the triage process. Issues related to reimbursement are discussed in a later section.

Principles of Effective Triage

- *Triage categories.* Problems may effectively be divided into those that require in-person evaluation immediately, in the near future, or not at all. Little pathology is missed when all patients are referred for immediate evaluation, but a different form of morbidity is created.

Good triage depends on the following factors:

- *Parent reliability and anxiety.* When a parent's description of an illness cannot be trusted because she is nervous, inarticulate, inexperienced, or unreliable, it is better to suggest early in-person evaluation of the patient. When the parent is deemed to be highly reliable, greater flexibility is appropriate.
- *Balanced waiting period.* Establishing a balanced waiting period

6

for a particular symptom depends on accessibility of medical care, time of day, and the potential seriousness of the complaint: A waiting period of 2 or 3 hours is reasonable before evaluating a nontoxic child with lower abdominal pain, but a much shorter waiting time should be used for a child who is febrile and lethargic.

- *Patient relations.* When a parent *believes* the situation to be an emergency, when possible, respond as though it is. When the parent *demands* an evaluation, make every effort to be accommodating; patient teaching can come later. When the parent makes frequent telephone calls for the same complaint, an in-person evaluation is usually in order.

Triage Techniques

- *Ask the most important questions first.* When there is an established policy to evaluate all febrile infants younger than 2 months old immediately, few other questions are necessary once it is learned that a 6-week-old baby has a rectal temperature of 101°F.
- *Narrow down the chief complaint.* Few parents offer a concise chief complaint over the phone such as "Two-year-old Jonny has had a cold and fever for 2 days and now says his left ear hurts." More commonly, a parent either describes each part of the child's anatomy in great detail and then recounts all previous ailments from the time of birth or offers as little information as possible, simply saying "Jonny is sick." The chief complaint can be narrowed down by responding with "I know he has been sick for some time. But I need to know what is bothering him right now."
- *Ask questions in symptom clusters.* Parents who offer little information can be helped along by asking questions in symptom groups rather than by asking about each symptom separately: "Does your daughter have a fever or a rash? Does she have a cough, cold, sore throat, or runny nose? Does she have vomiting, diarrhea, or stomach cramps?"

Diagnosing Illness

Although an accurate diagnosis is not usually necessary for good triage, a working, or *presumptive diagnosis* is needed before advice is offered. You should tell the parents that your diagnosis is tentative without sounding tentative yourself. This approach is more honest and has the advantage of allowing you to change your diagnosis with little or no embarrassment once the patient has been examined. You may find it useful to use phrases such as "I can't be certain without seeing your child, but the most likely cause of this problem is . . ." or "This illness does not sound serious. It may be necessary for me to see your child at a later time, but I'm reasonably certain that he has . . . ."

General
Principles

Common
Symptoms

Emergencies
and Traumas

Minor
Infections

Infectious
Diseases

Parenting
Concerns

Infant
Care

Screening Question Selectivity and Sensitivity

It is common to focus on screening questions that assess the most dominant symptoms. But those that evaluate the patient's general state of illness are often more helpful. One might be more concerned about a child with no fever who looks "toxic" than one with a high fever who is eating well, and playful. General screening questions are of two types: those that assess the *parent's anxiety level,* such as "Do you feel frightened about the way he looks?" and those that describe the child's general *medical condition,* such as "Does he look sicker than usual when he has a cold?" or "What has he been doing during the last hour?"

Practitioner's Bias

Most telephone calls are made to report common illnesses and common symptoms. Practitioners in a hospital setting and those who have just completed a residency or fellowship program may have an *illness-bias* because most of their patients are seriously ill and their training emphasizes complications of common and esoteric illnesses. Those practicing in an outpatient or office setting may be influenced more by a *wellness-bias* since the majority of their patients have more routine conditions.

Objectivity is difficult but essential. For example, the complaint "Mary is having trouble breathing" usually means she has a runny nose, and the statement "Jonny won't stop vomiting" usually means he has thrown up twice. A wellness-perception is more likely to be accurate, but one should not forget that the first patient may have bronchiolitis or have aspirated a peanut and the second might have early intestinal obstruction or encephalitis.

Likely Course of Illness

To avoid repeat calls advising you that symptoms have not yet resolved, whenever possible, tell parents the *expected duration* of the illness. It is surprising how many experienced parents sound astonished when they are told that their child's cold is contagious and will last 7 to 10 days. If you do not give a reminder, the chances of receiving a second call are quite good. Your discussion should also include the *period of contagion,* the *usual associated symptoms,* and the *activity level* allowed. These facts can be combined into a concise synoptic form based on your presumptive diagnosis. An example of a discussion regarding a 2-year-old's uncomplicated cold is as follows:

> It sounds to me as though Jonny has a simple cold. He may be a little irritable and eat less than usual during the next few days. He may also have a loose cough that is worse when he lies flat late both at night and in early morning. Many children with colds also develop some fever that can come and go during the entire 7 to 10 days of the runny nose.

He will be contagious to other children for about 1 week but can continue doing most activities if he feels well enough to do so. We usually don't prescribe cough and cold medicines for young children because they are not very effective and tend to make them even more cranky and irritable. But if your son seems uncomfortable from either fever or being stuffy, you might want to give him some acetaminophen or nose drops to help him feel better.

Prevalent Community Illness

Despite a normal reluctance to tell parents that an illness is "going around," it can be useful and desirable to do so. Parents are reassured to learn that other children in their neighborhood have similar symptoms. It is helpful for them to know that their child's fever and vomiting will probably last 1 day, followed by 2 days of diarrhea, and that deviant symptoms should be reported promptly. When herpangina is the prevalent community illness, reliable parents might initially be told to treat their children symptomatically unless they appear toxic or their symptoms persist longer than expected. When group A streptococcal illness is prevalent, it may be more appropriate to recommend that all patients with sore throats have throat cultures taken even when other symptoms are absent. Awareness of community illness can increase a practitioner's wellness-bias, however, and great care must be taken to rule out more serious conditions.

Treatment and Advice

Teaching Objectives
Telephone medicine is especially suited for achieving *short-term teaching objectives*: "Give Jonny one-half teaspoonful of medicine four times a day for the next 5 days. Don't give the medicine if it makes him irritable or causes him to have difficulty sleeping" or "Use a vaporizer when the heat is on in his room. But do not add any medicines to the water in the vaporizer's reservoir."

Long-term teaching objectives are better suited to office discussions. They usually gain better acceptance when mostly positive directives are used and negative directives are avoided. Negative suggestions frequently make the recipient want to perform the prohibition even more. When you read

STOP READING NOW

your first impulse is to continue reading to learn why you were told not to. Or you might continue reading because you feel antagonistic to the writer, or because you don't believe the author has the authority to tell you to stop. However, if the advice is presented as a *positive* suggestion, that it is in your best interest to stop reading, you might be more likely to comply. Well-phrased "suggestions" give the parent the feeling that he is the one who initiated the idea to stop. A more effective statement might be "Reading this small print can make your eyes feel very tired. You will feel more comfortable if you stop reading at this point and allow them to rest." Similarly, instead of saying, "Don't smoke when you have small children in the house," you might try using a more pragmatic suggestion, such as "When children live in a house with parents who smoke, they are much more likely to get colds, wheezing, and ear infections. If you stopped smoking it would be good for your children, but it might make you feel better too."

Organization

If you have trouble remembering what you want to say, imagine how difficult it is for a parent to remember your advice. Keep instructions as short and focused as possible, and put the most important and simple information first.

Teaching Aids

Teaching and motivational techniques used during telephone encounters are necessarily limited by time and lack of visual contact, but some of these strategies remain useful:

- Ask parents to *write down instructions.* The act of writing imprints information to memory and gives visual representation to what has been heard. Also the written note can be used for later reference.
- Have the caller *repeat instructions* after they have been given. This encourages last minute questions and makes misinterpretations less likely.
- Ask for *immediate feedback.* You might say "Is there anything that you don't understand or that we haven't covered?"
- Repeat important information. Using *different wording* may make it easier to understand and gives additional emphasis.

Prescribing Medicines

As with in-person patient contacts, the *risks and benefits* of prescribing medicines and treatments over the telephone should be carefully weighed before advice is given. In the past, practitioners have been reluctant to admit that they prescribed medicine over the phone, but it is obvious that *never* prescribing over the phone may create greater morbidity than it prevents and may delay appropriate treatment for recurrent illness or alleviation of a child's discomfort.

General principles to consider before prescribing treatments and medications over the telephone include the following.

- *Use available medications.* Ask which medicines are available in the home and which are already being given before suggesting an over-the-counter (OTC) or prescription remedy. It makes little sense for the parent to shop for a medication when a comparable substitute is already available.
- *Avoid masking symptoms.* Symptom-relieving medicines should be chosen to have the fewest side effects and to be least likely to mask symptoms or change laboratory values. One might prefer prescribing acetaminophen over the telephone to avoid lowering a sedimentation rate that might be obtained the following day.
- *Localized symptoms* are more amenable to telephone prescribing than are systemic symptoms.
- *Consider the age of the child.* The younger the patient, the more care should be taken before prescribing treatments or medicines without an examination.
- *Consider the general appearance of the child.* There is less risk when prescribing over the telephone for a child who appears well than for one who seems sick. The thought-provoking corollary is that it is safest to prescribe medicines for those patients least likely to need them.
- *Consider the names of medicines.* There is less confusion when prescribing medicines with the shortest brand names. Also ask the parents to write down the brand names before you spell them. It is surprising how few parents admit that they do not have a pencil until after instructions are given.
- *Avoid giving medicine when possible.* Parents sometimes forget that one reason for an examination is to *avoid* taking medicine unless it is needed. A parent requesting medication over the telephone often believes the practitioner to be oppositional when the request is refused. She can be pacified when the reason for refusal is presented as being in the child's and parent's best interest as by the statement "Erythromycin is the best antibiotic to give for bronchitis, but it commonly causes diarrhea and stomach cramps. I don't want to chance these additional symptoms unless I'm sure your child really needs it."
- *Interim prescription refills and dose changes may be warranted.* Telephoning medication changes and refills without having the patient's chart available for documentation and review creates obvious risks. However, when patients have "run out of medicine" for a chronic illness or clinical changes suggest that a change in medication or dosage is indicated, it is not always best to wait until regular office hours. To encourage parents to plan ahead, to improve documentation, and to avoid errors, *interim prescription* changes and refills can be made for small quantities with the un-

General Principles

Common Symptoms

Emergencies and Traumas

Minor Infections

Infectious Diseases

Parenting Concerns

Infant Care

derstanding that larger amounts will be prescribed during regular office hours when the chart is available.

Conclusion of the Call

When a parent hangs up the telephone she should have a general understanding of the nature of her child's symptoms, what treatment, if any, should be given for symptom relief, and under what circumstances she should call back the practitioner.

Call-Back Instructions
The initials "PCWAS" (remembered as Patient Conversation WAS) may be useful for outlining and documenting the elements of the concluding instructions: Parents should call for (P) *persistent,* (C) *changing* or new, (W) *worsening,* or (A) *anxiety*-provoking symptoms as well as those that are (S) *specific* to the child's illness.

Discharge instruction that might be given to a parent whose child has croup might be as follows.

> I want you to call me back if your daughter's breathing does not improve after sitting in a steamy bathroom for about 20 minutes (S). I also want you to call if she still sounds croupy by tomorrow morning (P), if any new or unusual symptoms develop during the night (C), if her breathing becomes more strained or labored (W), or if anything about her condition makes you feel nervous or upset (A).

Abandonment
Parents should feel that you will not desert them even though evening hours are approaching. Surprisingly, they are less likely to call back if they believe that you are nearby and accessible. Having immediate back-up increases confidence in their own judgment. You might say "If you need me tonight, please don't hesitate to call regardless of the hour."

Hidden Agendas
In addition to addressing the stated reason for a parent's call, it is also necessary to search for hidden agendas, *i.e.,* the stated reason for the call may not be the real reason it was made. Hidden agendas should be suspected when a call is made at an inappropriate time for the apparent severity of the complaint or when the degree of parental anxiety seems inappropriate to the problem. The most common example is when an experienced parent calls after hours to ask for the dose of a commonly used medicine. Rather than seeking advice, she is really calling "just to check in." She already knows the answer to her question but needs reassurance to be certain that what she was doing was right.

When hidden agendas are not addressed in a timely and complete manner, the parent will often be dissatisfied with the advice given and may call back in an irritated frenzy. For example, a mother calling late at night to learn whether her child's cold is contagious may really want to know whether she should cancel her elderly father's planned visit. A poorly timed call may also be made to settle angry spousal disputes: "I knew Sally was going to get a fever. I told you to call the doctor yesterday. Call him right now." Patients should be given the benefit of the doubt when calls seem inappropriate. It helps to maintain objectivity and politeness while evaluating the complaint (and can also preserve the clinician's sanity).

To sort out abusive calls from those with hidden agendas, the direct medical question should always be answered first, followed by the query "This is an awfully late hour to be calling about a simple cold. Is there a special reason you are calling now or is there something else that you need to know?" Firm discussions about appropriate times to call should be reserved for repeat offenders. Other parents will now be more reluctant to call after-hours unless it is medically necessary.

Phoning Ahead
If you believe that a patient should be examined in an emergency room and you will not be present at the patient's arrival, phone instructions ahead to that location. Parents are very appreciative when they are greeted by medical staff that expect them and already know about their child's problem. Give the probable diagnosis, suggested orders for treatment, and diagnostic tests that should be performed immediately.

Patient Transportation
In emergency situations, ask parents if they know how to get to the hospital or clinic and what type of transportation they will use. Instruct them to be cautious while driving and to have others drive them when possible. They may be extremely upset, and the trip to the hospital may become more dangerous than the actual illness. During a true emergency, give parents an ambulance or police telephone number, or you may wish to call for them.

Follow-up Calls
When you are concerned that a patient has a potentially serious illness, call the parent back a few hours later. You might have assumed that the child's condition improved, but the parent may have sought attention elsewhere. Even worse, he might not realize that the child's condition has been getting worse. Your call is never wasted. It is always appreciated by the parent and puts your mind at rest.

Common Symptoms

Emergencies and Traumas

Minor Infections

Infectious Diseases

Parenting Concerns

Infant Care

Improving Communication Skills

The first step toward improving communication skills is not taking them for granted.

Personal Style

Each practitioner should develop a style that reflects his or her unique personality. Some practitioners are more comfortable when they sound authoritarian; others work best using a casual style. No one technique works best for all clinicians, but flexibility is the key to achieving best overall success.

Telephone style should always sound personal. Even when calls are returned from a long list, the parent should be left with the impression that hers is the only call to be answered. In the same way that patients feel less rushed in an office setting when a practitioner is seated rather than standing, in telephone exchanges speaking slowly using a warm manner gives the impression that individual attention is being given to the call. With practice, one can become quite proficient at screening large numbers of calls without sounding hurried, mechanical, or disinterested. Instructions and questions should be crisp and precise, but the caller should feel that the practitioner is empathetic, knowledgeable, conscientious, and truly wants to help. Manner and voice must convey all of the feelings that would normally be projected by appearance.

Attitude

Many clinicians find that the most difficult transition when moving from a training program into a practice setting is getting used to the conflict of being "off" (not in the office) and being "on" (on call) at the same time. Intrusive telephone calls during hectic office hours can be managed effectively with the aid of ancillary personnel. But an unending flow of telephone calls interrupting family time or simply during eating may transform each call into a personal affront. The child's parents usually determine the timing of the call, and the potential for annoyance increases proportionately to the size of the practice. Each patient can become an

Common Symptoms

Emergencies and Traumas

Minor Infections

Infectious Diseases

Parenting Concerns

Infant Care

Jeffrey L. Brown: *Pediatric Telephone Medicine: Principles, Triage, and Advice,* Second Edition. Copyright © 1994 J. B. Lippincott Company

15

General
Principles

Common
Symptoms

Emergencies
and Traumas

Minor
Infections

Infectious
Diseases

Parenting
Concerns

Infant
Care

unwanted visitor into the physician's home, and personality, fatigue, and general attitude can strongly influence the quality of response made to the call.

Empathy

It is easier to gain patients' trust when they feel that you relate to them. Matching your level of interest and concern with theirs helps give them the feeling that you are both "in synch." Matching emotional level and tone are only some of the pacing methods that can be used. *Stating the obvious* also helps to establish a bond between you and the caller. This can be accomplished by saying "Mrs. Smith, you sound very upset," or "When you called last night, you sounded frightened. Until you get used to them, each of Cathy's wheezing attacks can be very disturbing." Your observation tells her that you are interested in her as well her daughter's illness, that you have noticed her emotional state, and that you are not judgmental of her. If it is necessary to remind her that she overreacted to a particular situation, do so only after the medical problem has been carefully discussed and resolved.

Stating the obvious makes your observations similar to those the parent made and gives you something in common. If you can also offer a *compliment,* all the better. An appropriate response might be "The last time you were in the office I was very impressed by the way that your children behaved." It has often been said that "flattery will get you everywhere." We all enjoy being noticed—especially with approval.

Language

It is impolite to use language that your patient is not likely to understand, and the results can be disastrous. Speaking a foreign language to someone who doesn't understand is foolish and a waste of time; using medical terminology rather than common everyday terms is not very different. Medical jargon used comfortably with colleagues may be impossible for patients to decipher. Easy to understand terms do not lower patients' opinions of you; they will love you for it. Don't call a cut a laceration or refer to drawing blood as performing a venipuncture. Such communication is thoughtless and becomes a barrier to providing good care.

It is also necessary to develop a vocabulary of descriptive terms for physical signs that create a visual image for the caller. When there is concern about labored breathing, for example, one might ask if the child "has a heaving chest or has to pull or strain to breathe."

16

Being a Good Listener

If you don't hear the parent's question or answer, you can't give a proper response. It frustrates parents when your answer suggests that you were not listening to them. If your mind does wander, apologize. Say "I'm really sorry. I know that you just told me, but what medicine did you say your daughter was taking for her cough?"

A variation of this theme is answering a question before it has been asked, as in saying "I know you're wondering why I am in the office now, but I decided to come in to do some paperwork." The only thing the parent is wondering is why you told him that.

Being a Good Questioner

Special effort must be taken to avoid "leading" parents into giving specific answers; they may believe that you will be annoyed or disappointed if they don't answer as expected. Also the information you receive may not be accurate. Questions of this type often end with ". . . aren't you?" or "Isn't that true?" as in the statements "You are very nervous about this, aren't you?" or "You haven't been happy since you have moved here. Isn't that true?" It is preferable to ask questions that allow *any* answer to be given comfortably. More general questions might be "Have you been feeling nervous or upset about this?" or "How have things been going since you moved to this area?"

Focused but open-ended questions can still allow the parent room to answer. An example of this sort of question is "The last few times I saw you, you seemed very nervous and upset. How do you feel today?"

Telephone Record Keeping and Liability

Documentation

Medical Reasons for Documentation

Documentation is useful as an organizational aid for tracking a patient's illness patterns and making treatment decisions. Patient management information should be recorded in the permanent record whenever possible. This includes:

- *Medications.* Both prescription and over-the-counter medicines that are prescribed, discontinued, or changed in dosage, as well as adverse reactions to them.
- *Nonroutine illnesses injuries or symptoms.* Advice and treatment for conditions that have the potential for complications or unfavorable outcome.
- *Referrals.* Referrals made for diagnostic tests or consultations.
- *Test results and recommendations.* Telephoned test results and telephoned recommendations made by consultants.

- *Pertinent parental perceptions and actions.* Advice and recommendations made by staff that are refused by caretakers, especially when there is refusal to bring the child for an immediate evaluation. Other actions or inactions that you believe not to be in the child's best interest should also be recorded, such as administration of home remedies that may be harmful.

Other Reasons for Documentation

- *Liability.* When documentation is made for reasons of potential liability, there may be a bonus in improved record quality since legal considerations often parallel those of good care. But fear of malpractice actions may result in documentation that is wasteful of time and creates a false sense of security. By necessity, after-hours telephone encounters usually occur without referring to the patient's chart, and when calls are answered while physicians are performing examinations and other patient-related activities, chart access is often difficult or impractical. It is unrealistic to expect that all calls will receive complete documentation in a busy pediatric practice, and a constant effort must be made to balance pragmatics with medical need.

Jeffrey L. Brown: *Pediatric Telephone Medicine: Principles, Triage, and Advice,*
Second Edition. Copyright © 1994 J. B. Lippincott Company

General
Principles

Common
Symptoms

Emergencies
and Traumas

Minor
Infections

Infectious
Diseases

Parenting
Concerns

Infant
Care

- *Personal comfort.* Clinicians must find a level of documentation consistent with their personal comfort level but should also have an awareness of their motivation when making documenting decisions. In an effort to "ward off the evil spirit," some practitioners feel the need to record everything regardless of practicality or necessity: "The more I write, the better the doctor I become." Others may use denial to justify poor record keeping: "The less I write, the less chance this encounter will have a bad outcome."

Recording Telephone Messages

Even with the best intent, intense telephone traffic may result in occasional unrecorded telephone contacts and misplaced or erroneous messages. Some methods for improving documentation and reducing error are listed below.

- *Telephone logs books* with carbonless-copy paper or carbon sheets. The minimum information to be recorded on each sheet should include the patient's name, age, and chief complaint, the person for whom the call is intended, the time and date the call was received, the parent's call-back number, and the disposition to the call when appropriate.
- *Stickers* are useful for recording after-hours calls that are to be entered into the chart at a later time.
- *Telephone answering service logs* will often be mailed or faxed to the office on request. Pertinent entries can then be charted daily or weekly after review by the physician, or the original log can be stored for later reference.
- *Patient reporting* of events is an excellent way to provide backup to usual documenting practices. It can be especially useful when the practitioner wishes to document after-hours calls but will not be present in the office the following day. Patients can be instructed to telephone the office during regular hours to tell the nurse or secretary to record pertinent events into the chart. These might include tetanus toxoid administered in an emergency room, a presumed allergic reaction to an antibiotic, or a rash suggestive of chickenpox. It is also helpful to instruct parents to call after they have consulted with a doctor to whom they were referred or to report that a diagnostic test has been scheduled or has been performed.

Limitations of Good Documentation

As is true of office visit notes, the completeness of documentation for telephone encounters usually depends on the potential seriousness of the complaint. Unfortunately, the complaint may not appear serious until it

General
Principles

Common
Symptoms

Emergencies
and Traumas

Minor
Infections

Infectious
Diseases

Parenting
Concerns

Infant
Care

is examined retrospectively. A well-documented note may provide some protection from criticism, but "He said . . . ," "She said . . ." situations commonly arise regardless of what is written in the chart. The telephone record of a child later diagnosed with epiglottitis might read "Croupy cough for 1 hr. No URI, temp or significant dyspnoea. To call for worsening symptoms. Rx Steam." But after a frantic trip to the hospital, the mother might confuse statements she made to the emergency room physician a few hours later with those given to the doctor when she first called. "I told that doctor my child looked sicker than I have ever seen her look before." And if the statement had actually been made at the time of the call, the doctor might say that he did not record it because the mother also described the child as looking "alert, playful, and having good color."

Commonly reported complaints seen with routine illnesses such as fever, feeding poorly, sleeping a lot, looking pale, and vomiting offer little protection when they have been noted in the chart but the child is later diagnosed as having meningitis. And in some cases they might even be used to suggest that evaluation of the child should have been more aggressive: Many children who have bacterial meningitis will have presenting symptoms of fever and vomiting, but few children with fever and vomiting will have bacterial meningitis as the cause. Also there is no way to document a call that was never received but that a parent says was made in January 5 years earlier: "I called twice, but nobody called me back." Even better than average telephone logging systems do not always reflect calls that are put through directly to the doctor or nurse, and few practitioners can testify that *every* call gets recorded.

Even more disturbing are those instances when *excessive documentation* can prove harmful to a malpractice defense. Consider the mother who reports that her son sustained what appeared to be minor head trauma. Time was taken to document the warning to watch for an altered state of consciousness, nausea, vomiting, incoordination, and worsening headache, but no mention was made of a warning about abnormal gait, slurred speech, bruising behind an ear, or discharge from an ear or nostril. Risk of litigation might *increase* if these signs or symptoms are ignored by the parent since their absence from the documented call-back instructions is now highlighted.

Limited Documentation with "PCWAS"
Even when there has been *no documentation* of a call, a credible defense can still be made if the practitioner can honestly say that "It is my usual and customary practice to give complete instructions to every parent who telephones with this complaint. When an examination does not seem to be necessary, I tell every parent who reports head trauma to call me back if the child develops a severe headache, persistent vomiting, or difficul-

General Principles

Common Symptoms

Emergencies and Traumas

Minor Infections

Infectious Diseases

Parenting Concerns

Infant Care

ty staying awake. I also tell them to call if even minor symptoms continue, if they seem to be getting worse, if there are any new or unusual findings, or if anything about the child's condition makes the parent feel nervous. I don't document every call, especially when it has been made for a common symptom or a minor injury. The absence of a documenting note in this case suggests that this incident did not sound serious when it was presented to me." The strength of such a claim might be increased when a telephone triage manual has been accepted as part of the office guidelines.

One should consider whether *limited documentation* that includes the "PCWAS" call-back abbreviation (Persistent, Changing, Worsening, Anxiety-causing or Specific symptoms) might provide a reasonable compromise for recording the pertinent medical facts of most calls with a minimal expenditure of time. The telephone contact described above might have been documented as "Mom reports minor head trauma with minimal symptoms. Told to call for PCWAS." (See p. 12).

Delayed Documentation
Erroneous interpretation of calls made just prior to the diagnosis of a serious illness can be minimized when their content is recorded as part of the patient's *history of present illness.* Such documentation in the office, emergency room, or inpatient hospital chart can be very useful even when its importance is not immediately obvious. Rules for documentation include:
- *Dating.* The note should be dated for the time it is *actually* written.
- *Content.* The note should include the time of the call, who initiated it, what was said by both parties, and its eventual disposition. Other pertinent information includes social history, consultants who were called, and medicines that were administered.
- *Chart uniformity.* A note may have its authenticity questioned when it uses a format different from others in the chart. If call-back instructions have never been recorded for other previous illnesses, documentation of instructions given just prior to a hospitalization for a ruptured appendix may seem suspicious. *A previously entered chart note should never be altered or amended* unless the following rules are observed: Entries requiring correction can be crossed out with a single line so that the original entry remains legible; correction fluid should never be used. And notes may have additions made if the time and date of the addition is clearly recorded.

Incorporating previous telephone conversations into the history of present illness creates excellent documentation for the most important calls. An office chart note made to record a simple illness might read, "Mother called to report mild URI yesterday. Now the patient has right ear pain and temp of 103°F since early AM." The *admission note* for a child hospitalized with meningitis might read:

> This 3-year-old male was in previously good health until early yesterday morning when his mother noted fever without other symptoms. She called my office at 3 P.M. to report a temperature of 102°F after administration of acetaminophen. He was said to not appear especially ill and had eaten both breakfast and lunch. She was told to call for localizing or worsening symptoms. Following a service call at 9:30 P.M., she stated that he had passed a few loose stools and vomited twice. His general condition was said to be unchanged. The mother was told to offer only clear liquids until morning and to use acetaminophen rectal suppositories prn. She was instructed to call back if the child appeared to be worsening, developed severe abdominal pain, or if she was concerned about his general appearance. At 6 A.M. today she called through the service to report that his rectal temperature was now 104°F and that he seemed very lethargic. I told her to bring him directly to the emergency room for an immediate examination. She did not arrive until nearly 2 hours later, stating that she did not want to leave her new infant at home alone. At examination this child was febrile, extremely lethargic, and had nuchal rigidity. A lumbar puncture revealed cloudy fluid. At 8:45 A.M. I telephoned Dr. M. R. Ivey, a pediatric neurologist, who recommended stat administration of the following medications:. . . .

If this same child was admitted to the hospital by someone else, a documenting note describing previous telephone calls can be entered as a *progress note* the first time the child is visited at the hospital, or an entry can be made into the patient's *office chart,* being certain that it is dated for the time it is actually written. "Patient admitted to Community Hospital early yesterday morning with a presumptive diagnosis of pneumococcal meningitis. The mother first called me 2 days ago at 3 P.M. to report. . . ." If medical complications follow this illness, years later it may be otherwise impossible to remember who called whom and at what hour. There may also be some value to placing copies of the answering service and office telephone logs in the patient's chart or flagging them for later reference. Calls regarding serious illness but not requiring hospitalization can also be made as delayed office chart notations if proper rules of entry are followed.

Common Symptoms

Emergencies and Traumas

Minor Infections

Infectious Diseases

Parenting Concerns

Infant Care

23

Telephone Liability

The Doctor–patient Relationship

Once a doctor–patient relationship has been established, the potential liability incurred during telephone contacts is similar to that during patient visits. When telephoned advice is offered regarding a child's probable diagnosis, treatment, or need for examination, a doctor–patient relationship may have been created even though the clinician has never met the parents or examined the patient. "These symptoms sound as though your child might have pneumonia. I think you should bring her to the hospital emergency room to have some X-rays taken."

No such relationship would generally be considered to exist if a new patient is referred directly to a hospital emergency room or clinic for medical care as a *statement of policy* without commenting on the child's condition. Some confusion can be avoided when the clinician's future role in the child's care is clearly stated at the time of the parent's call, as in the following exchange: "My daughter has had a fever and cough for the past 2 days." "I'm sorry, but our office is not accepting new patients at the present time and we will not be able to take care of your daughter. If you believe the problem is urgent, you can bring her directly to the emergency room to be seen by one of the hospital physicians. If it is not urgent, the hospital medical staff office can supply you with the names of other physicians in our community."

Why Parents Initiate Malpractice Actions

To avoid malpractice actions, it is helpful to first recognize factors that may motivate parents to initiate a complaint against a practitioner. These include:

- *Expectation.* When parents expect a favorable medical outcome because of actual or implied statements made by the clinician, they may be more likely to assume that an error in management was made if complications arise.
- *Investigation.* When there is uncertainty as to whether poor practice procedures have taken place, a malpractice action may be initiated to allow an outside party to evaluate the treatment that was rendered.
- *Establishing blame.* Like health-care professionals, parents often perform a soul-searching review of events that occurred prior to a bad outcome that followed their child's illness. They may question whether they should have reported the illness in a more timely manner, described symptoms differently, or if alternate treatment should have been sought. When the practitioner is shown to be at fault, parents may feel less guilty about their role as it related to this illness.

24

- *Retribution.* When parents believe their child has been injured because of bad medical practice, they might wish to punish the practitioner for the perceived wrong.
- *Remuneration.* Occasionally, parents bring suit for personal gain. More commonly, they may believe it to be their parental responsibility to obtain any compensation possible to protect their injured child from future financial burdens that might result from the illness or condition.
- *Institutionalization.* In a litigious environment, parents are sometimes told by others that they would be "foolish" if they did not bring suit following a poor medical outcome. After all, they may reason, "it doesn't really affect the doctor; it is the insurance company that would have to pay."

Strategies To Avoid Malpractice Actions
- *Practice good medicine.* It is extremely unfortunate when clinicians are named as defendants in malpractice actions even though they followed proper and acceptable procedure, but there is little defense when bad medical practices are responsible for a poor patient outcome.
- *Document telephone calls.* It is sometimes said that a good practitioner should document everything. "If you didn't write it, you didn't do it." Recording pertinent facts can be a valuable aid to providing good medical care to the patient; it may also be helpful to avoid litigation. But complete recording of all events is not usually practical, and even when documentation is present, negative interpretation of the documenting notes may limit their effectiveness.
- *Avoid ambiguities.* Ambiguous or incomplete statements can lead to misunderstandings, with disastrous results. Avoiding ambiguity requires a constant process of refinement. Following each telephone contact, the clinician should rethink questions asked and instructions given to determine whether different language might have lessened the possibility of misunderstandings. Special attention should be given to those conversations in which it was obvious that a missed communication took place.

    Even in the best of circumstances, parents' recollections and interpretations of conversations can be selective. Consider the instruction "This sounds like a simple and routine condition; I don't think there is any need to worry. However, if your son's illness does not improve by tomorrow, if it seems to be getting worse, or if there are any changes that make you feel nervous about him, there might be a more serious problem and you should call me back." Many parents will have accurate recall, but others will have different interpretations of what was said. Some will call back one-

Common Symptoms

Emergencies and Traumas

Minor Infections

Infectious Diseases

Parenting Concerns

Infant Care

General
Principles

Common
Symptoms

Emergencies
and Traumas

Minor
Infections

Infectious
Diseases

Parenting
Concerns

Infant
Care

half hour later to report "He looks fine. But you said this could be serious and I should call you back," while others might say "He became much sicker after we spoke, but I didn't call back because you said this wasn't serious and there was no need to worry."

- *Avoid creating parental guilt.* When there has been a delay in diagnosis or treatment because of parental inaction, evaluate and treat the medical problem immediately but avoid the temptation to accuse parents of incompetence or neglect. Increasing parental anxiety and guilt instantly create a hostile relationship. It is a poor strategy to say "This child is very ill. You should have called me sooner. Now I can't guarantee how this will come out." Paradoxically, parents might be more likely to blame a bad outcome on medical management than on their delay in seeking treatment when they feel that the clinician is judgmental of them. Such considerations need not preclude empathetic but necessary fact finding and parent teaching, which can be conveyed by saying "This child looks as though he may have been sick for some time. I know it can be very difficult to evaluate an illness like this at home. We can talk about that later. Let me get started on his treatment right away. I want to do the very best I can for your son."

- *Create realistic expectations.* At times of serious illness, avoid the temptation to say "Everything will turn out all right" when you are not sure it will. Instead, try using "Your daughter has an illness that is potentially very serious. Many children with this problem do well with early treatment. Let's hope that she falls into that group."

- *Be aware of a wellness-bias.* Abdominal pain is only infrequently caused by appendicitis, or headaches by brain tumors. Clinicians in tertiary care centers may have a bias toward unusual and complicated illness, but those in a typical practice setting know that few of the children seen will have other than routine problems. *Wellness-bias* is made worse when many other children in the community have similar symptoms and when the patient has been examined in the recent past. One must be extremely cautious when saying "Fever with vomiting is going around," or "Of course he still has pain. I just saw him 2 hours ago and he has only taken one dose of medicine." Because the clinician cannot visualize the child during the conversation, each telephone encounter should "stand alone" with only limited importance placed on a recent examination or telephone conversation about this illness. "When I saw your child 2 hours ago he didn't seem very sick. I told you he might not be better until morning. Is there anything about his condition that changed to make you call back so soon?"

- *Trust your instincts.* "Intuition" about a telephone conversation combines a clinician's previous experience, level of expertise, knowledge of prevalent community illnesses, reliability of the parent, temperament of the child, and strengths and weaknesses of the medical facility. It is not unusual for intuitive feelings to be more reliable than the formal presentation of symptoms.
- *Be accommodating.* When parents demand an immediate examination for their child, their request should be granted whenever possible. They may be expressing anxiety about the child's condition that they cannot otherwise put into words. Similarly, when multiple calls about the same condition are received during a short period of time, an examination should be arranged as soon as is practical.
- *When in doubt, examine the patient.* Visual inspection is a clinician's best tool for assessing the seriousness of an illness. The child's appearance must be relayed by proxy during telephone contacts, and history taking cannot always substitute for a physical examination. When significant doubt exists about the possibility of serious illness, the child should be examined.

Staff Liability

Depending on the practice setting, the physician in charge may be held personally liable for advice or triage given by staff members. At a minimum, there is a responsibility to assure that staff are aware of practice policy. Nurses and other professionals or paraprofessionals may be instructed to provide parents with well-child guidance, treatment advice for common symptoms, and in some cases telephone evaluation of more complex conditions. But anyone who answers the phone performs patient triage when he or she decides whether the doctor should be called immediately or if the call-back can be delayed until the doctor returns from the hospital or finishes examining patients.

From the time of employment, staff members should have a clear understanding of the kind of advice they are allowed to offer, preferred advice for common symptoms, and practice triage guidelines. For purposes of liability, it is useful to have printed materials modified or used directly from a triage manual such as this one and a receptionist's handbook that outlines specific office policy. These guidelines should be subjected to physician review and updated regularly. Staff members can sign or otherwise indicate that they have read the protocols; they should be asked for their own input; and telephone-related problems should be discussed at staff meetings. In some settings, role play and other teaching techniques for common or serious complaints may be useful.

General
Principles

Common
Symptoms

Emergencies
and Traumas

Minor
Infections

Infectious
Diseases

Parenting
Concerns

Infant
Care

Patient Confidentiality

Medical information about a patient should not be released to others without the consent of the child's guardian, most usually a parent. Errors in confidentiality are commonly made when well-meaning clinicians or staff try to be helpful to the patient or family. It must be remembered that the caller may not be who she says she is and may not have information about the patient's condition specifically because the parents don't want her to have it. Similarly, the person who says he is a representative from a family's insurance company really may be trying to obtain information for an unauthorized third party.

Insurance company inquiries are rarely emergencies, and it is not necessary to respond to them until the identity and authority of the caller is clearly established. Staff should be especially wary when answering queries that pertain to a patient's *prior illness* or to a current or previous *accidental injury*. The best defense against unauthorized release of information is to maintain a high degree of suspicion and to discuss this issue frequently at staff meetings. When the caller is not known personally or there is uncertainty about the purpose for the call, the response can sound polite and helpful without confidential information being supplied. Consider these inquiries and their appropriate responses:

Hello. My name is Doctor Harris. I am the grandfather of little Jonny Harris. I understand that you admitted him to the Intensive Care Unit at Community Hospital yesterday. I'm very worried about him. Can you please tell me how he is doing?

I am very anxious to discuss Jonny's admission with you, but you realize that I can't give you any information about him until I have permission from his dad. Please have your son call me and I will be happy to tell you anything you would like to know. In the meantime, I can tell you that he is getting excellent care and that his condition is stable. I'm sorry I can't be of more help right now. Give me your telephone number and I'll get right back to you as soon as I receive your son's call.

Hello. I am calling for the Peoples' National Health Insurance Company. John Harris was involved in an automobile accident yesterday. He is insured by our company. Can you please tell me the extent of his injuries and how long you expect him to remain in the hospital?

I'm sorry but we can't release that information without his parents' consent. Please give me your name, telephone number, and their policy number. We will get back to you as soon as possible.

Hello. Mrs. Harris told me that her son John Harris is a patient of yours. I am a close friend of their family, but I haven't been able to get in touch with her since they moved 6 months ago. I have some very important papers that I need to mail to her. Could you please give me Mrs. Harris's address and telephone number?

I'm sorry but our office can't give out personal information about our patients or their families. If you leave your name and number, we will call Mrs. Harris and pass your message along to her.

When there is an extenuating circumstance and you believe the caller must be given information immediately, you may wish to follow these rules:
- Insist on calling the caller back to validate the telephone number, or use an electronic device to determine the caller's number.
- Once contacted, tell the parents what information was given and explain why you felt that you could not wait for their approval.
- Document the entire incident in the patient's chart.

General Principles

Common Symptoms

Emergencies and Traumas

Minor Infections

Infectious Diseases

Parenting Concerns

Infant Care

Practical Considerations

Common
Symptoms

Emergencies
and Traumas

Minor
Infections

Infectious
Diseases

Parenting
Concerns

Infant
Care

Volume of Telephone Calls

Good practice management can go a long way toward training parents to
telephone during regular hours, but a busy pediatric practice should expect a high volume of calls both during and after-hours. The volume of
ill-timed calls can remain quite high even when only a small percentage
of parents chronically telephone for trivial advice: If a practice contains
1000 families with 2000 children, and each family makes only 2 "unnecessary" after-hours calls a year, there will be an average of 5 "unnecessary" calls per day; and if only 1 or 2 percent of the children have medical complaints at any given time, another 40 "appropriate" calls per day
might be received. It should be no surprise that a physician covering a
three- or four-doctor group during a winter weekend might therefore be
answering telephone calls all day long.

Types of Telephone Calls

Most telephone calls received concerning illness are made for relatively
few symptoms: Fever, upper respiratory symptoms, vomiting, rash, and
trauma are among the most common. The types of calls received vary depending on the patient population, the time of day, the season, and the
practice setting. It is helpful to review telephone logs to categorize calls
received at your location and to emphasize the most common complaints
when reviewing symptomatic advice and triage instructions with staff.

Telephone Calling Patterns

The time of day when calls are received can provide a clue to evaluating
the degree and type of problem. It is also helpful when searching for hidden agendas:

- *Early morning* calls are often made for illness that has been present throughout the night. These callers may have been caring for
  ill children without sleep for many hours. They expect and often
  deserve early morning appointments when possible.

Jeffrey L. Brown: *Pediatric Telephone Medicine: Principles, Triage, and Advice,*
Second Edition. Copyright © 1994 J. B. Lippincott Company

31

- *Late afternoon* calls may reflect illness that began while children were in school. Parents may not learn of symptoms until the children return home or are sent home by the school nurse; working mothers may not learn about the illness until the child is picked up from day-care or from the baby-sitter.

- *Early evening* calls are frequently made by parents whose children have been sick all day. But the call is not made until one parent arrives home from work and intimidates the other by saying, "Why didn't you tell the doctor about Jimmy's illness sooner?" Early evening is an especially stressful time for parents of young children. Typically, the children are tired, bored, and hungry; dinner is being prepared; and the homecoming of one or both parents is disruptive to the child's routine. Everyone may be generally irritable, making this a common time for calls about accidental injuries.

- *Late evening* calls (10:00 to 11:30 P.M.) are often received from parents whose children have been sick for more than a few hours but who are now apprehensive for fear that they will be left without medical advice as the night progresses. In addition to displaying those symptoms likely to worsen at night, such as coughing, wheezing and fever, children may appear more ill at night because daytime distractions are absent.

- *Friday afternoon* calls concerning routine illness may increase when parents are worried that weekend plans will be ruined or that medical attention may not readily be available. Allowance should be made for these not so unreasonable concerns, and criteria for examination should be liberalized.

- *Weekend* calls after office hours can be weather-dependent. On sunny days and during summertime, parents take children on outings despite the presence of moderate illness and are likely to call on returning to report that their child has been sick all day. They may also call Sunday night to ask if the child can be sent to school the next morning. When there is inclement weather, calls may be made all through the weekend day because attention is now focused on the sick child at home, and there is a tendency to seek help more quickly.

Telephone Calling Hours

The *advantages* of scheduled telephone calling hours include the need to answer fewer calls while examining patients and parental reassurance by your advertised availability. The *disadvantages* include long waiting times and busy signals during the calling hours because of limited access, the possibility that the practitioner may not be available when treating emergencies, and the likelihood that scheduled times encourage calls about trivial concerns.

One solution is to have *preferred calling times* for parents to make calls for well-child advice, laboratory results, and appointments. It is best to suggest preferred calling times that are not during hours of greatest telephone traffic. The receptionist can then triage calls depending upon urgency. When it is expected that the practitioner will not call back immediately or within one-half hour, parent dissatisfaction can be greatly reduced when he or she is told the most likely time that the call-back will be made. This thoughtful advice avoids having parents who have waited anxiously at the phone for hours greet the caller with an angry "What would have happened if my child had had a *real* emergency?"

Training Patients

Telephone policy should be discussed with parents when they first enter the practice—while teaching new baby care or at the time of the child's first physical examination. Printed office policy forms that include a section on telephone calling preferences can be very helpful (p. 285). No matter how intense your effort, some parents will regularly call at their convenience rather than attempt to comply with your office schedule. They should be made to feel that you are providing a 24-hour service but that it is to *their* advantage to try to limit contacts to office hours. You can explain "If you have an emergency you can call at any time. But when the call is not urgent we would like you to call during regular office hours. That way your child's chart is available to us if we need it."

Responding to After-hours Calls

Parents are frequently unaware that their child's physician may not *want* to talk with them after-hours, either because they consider the doctor to be a personal friend or because they believe that all physicians *should* provide 24-hour service. Pediatricians and family practitioners have both the advantage and disadvantage of dispensing primary care and are often first in line when parents seek the answer to a medical question. When a child develops a postoperative complication or traumatizes a tooth, the pediatrician will often receive the first phone call because the parent "didn't want to bother" the surgeon or the dentist.

The attitude clinicians assume toward after-hours calls often determines personal happiness and can greatly affect practice growth. There is real consolation in knowing that most patient calls *are* justified either

33

General Principles

Common Symptoms

Emergencies and Traumas

Minor Infections

Infectious Diseases

Parenting Concerns

Infant Care

for medical or psychological reasons and that giving a helpful response to an after-hours call can greatly alleviate parental anxiety or patient discomfort. Most importantly, the telephoned contact may result in early treatment of a seriously ill child.

Pharmacy Liaison

The pharmacist should be considered an essential team member for effective telephone patient management. Compile an easily accessible list of the most frequently used pharmacy phone numbers and learn pharmacies' policies and hours of operation. If the pharmacies in your area use a rotation for weekend and holiday coverage, request a copy of their schedule and keep it at appropriate locations.

Whenever possible, try to visit the pharmacies you deal with on a regular basis. The pharmacist's help can make your job easier and more effective. When pharmacists think of you as a person rather than as a voice on the phone, they are more responsive. They are also a frequent source of referrals, and many have a long-term knowledge of the families that they service. Most importantly, they screen your prescriptions for accuracy before they are dispensed.

Hospitalized Patients

Telephone techniques for communicating with hospital staff are learned by the practitioner as a house officer. But few practitioners develop the habit of calling parents who are at the bedside of hospitalized patients. Parents are reassured and appreciative when their doctor asks to talk with them when checking on the child's progress with the nurse. Changes in condition and errors in management are often described by parents that were not passed on by the professional staff. As an added bonus, these calls may save an unnecessary trip back to the child's bedside late in the day. When the physician makes daily rounds on maternity floors, new mothers may not always be available if they are receiving nursing care or are in the shower. Again, a reassuring phone call later that morning may sometimes be preferable to waiting for the mothers to return to bed.

Follow-up to Office Visits

Telephone contacts can be used in a manner similar to follow-up office visits by instructing parents to telephone 24 or 48 hours after a visit *regardless* of the *child's condition,* but sooner if necessary. These telephoned follow-ups are especially useful for conditions not likely to be progressive but that have the potential for significant complications, *e.g.,* minimal wheezing or early swelling of an eyelid. In some cases, it might be best to maintain a checklist to be certain that these call-backs have been made.

Billing for Telephone Time

Professional advice given over the telephone should be reimbursed at the same rate as in-person services. But, because clinicians do not traditionally charge on a strict time-for-service schedule, there has been a reluctance to bill for telephone time. Those providing telephone services through managed care networks should make every effort to negotiate an appropriate fee schedule for telephone time: Telephoned advice is less expensive than office or follow-up patient visits. Professionals treating patients on a *fee-for-service* basis must consider whether the costs of paperwork and billing for telephone time make this practice worthwhile or whether compensation should be received by *incorporating fees* into charges for office visits according to the following formula:

(hourly rate × telephone hours) ÷ (number of patient visits per day) = increased charge for each patient visit

For example, a practitioner generating $100 per hour while seeing 20 patients a day might increase the charge for each office visit by $5 if 1 hour per day is spent on the telephone. Newly diagnosed diabetics, homebound patients confined to bed, and others requiring frequent telephoned consultations should have billing arrangements for this telephone time *agreed upon in advance.*

Salaried physicians and those working within systems that pay for services on a capitation basis receive *reversed reimbursement* for telephone time, that is, office efficiency and profits increase when telephone consultations effectively decrease in-person visits.

Telephone Equipment

Home and office telephone equipment deserves as much attention as other medical apparatus to be used on a daily basis. The practice setting and patient volume determine the type of equipment needed, but the following considerations should be noted.

- *Expansion.* Choose a telephone system that can be expanded to accept a greater number of lines in the future.
- *Number of lines.* Even a solo practitioner should have at least two lines designated for incoming calls from patients and two "pri-

General
Principles

Common
Symptoms

Emergencies
and Traumas

Minor
Infections

Infectious
Diseases

Parenting
Concerns

Infant
Care

vate" lines designated for outgoing calls and emergency incoming calls such as those from the hospital. One incoming line should "jump" to the second incoming line, and private lines should also jump one to the other.

- *Office intercom.* The telephone system can be used as an office intercom, but care must be taken to assure that private messages not be communicated into patient areas. An appropriate intercom message might be "Miss Jones, please pick up on intercom" rather than "Miss Jones, please make an appointment for Susan Henderson. She is on line 2. She has been bleeding again."

- *Music and message on hold.* To assure parents that they have not been cut off when they are placed on hold, many offices use equipment that plays recorded music or informational messages. These can discuss office policy or provide health or parenting tips; tapes can be made in-house or professionally prepared in either "packaged" or personalized formats. Before playing radio station music over your system, consider patient annoyance at listening to commercials and discuss the legality of doing so with an attorney.

- *Optional equipment.* Choosing "bells and whistles" for your telephone system can best be done with the help of a consultant. Useful options include memory dialing, automatic redial, lightweight headsets to free the hands of the receptionist, and speaker phones that double as intercoms.

- *Home telephones.* Home telephones should have plentiful extensions with a separate line (and possibly call waiting) dedicated solely to professional use. Many practitioners find that using a phone next to the bed with a lighted handset dial is helpful when making and answering calls in the middle of the night.

- *Telephone service.* Carefully check the references of the company selling you equipment and service. The company's reputation for reliability may be even more important than system cost or the equipment that you buy.

- *Portable phones.* Car and portable phones were once thought to be an extravagance but should now be considered a necessity for any practitioner who must answer emergency calls. Improvement in lifestyle from increased mobility and decreased anxiety more than compensates for any added business expense.

- *Credit card calls.* Credit card calls avoid the need to carry loose change when pay phones must be used. Establishing a professional credit card number should receive early priority even when it must be paid for out of pocket.

- *Paging devices.* Paging devices that display the number to be called decrease calls to the answering service. But when a page is not received because the number has been entered improperly, the pager is out of range, or there is a mechanical malfunction, it may take longer for the problem to be discovered. Having all calls and responses to them documented by your service can be an asset for decreasing liability and monitoring practice efficiency.

- *Voice-mail systems.* Some answering services provide voice-mail services. These may be useful in some limited settings and for specialty group practices. The voice-mail menu must be carefully constructed and reviewed at regular intervals to reduce patient confusion and to highlight instructions for talking to a "live person" when there is an emergency. Even when these systems are effective, parents may perceive them to be impersonal and may have difficulty using them when they are nervous.

- *Recorded messages.* Recorded messages are an effective way to decrease after-hours calls. An answering machine or in some cases an answering service voice-mail system may be used. The recording should be less than 30 seconds in duration. An example of a message suitable for general pediatric practice is as follows:

    You have reached the pediatric offices of Drs. Alpha, Bravo, and Charlie. Our regular office hours are 9 A.M. to 5 P.M. weekdays and 9 A.M. to 12 noon on Saturdays, Sundays, and holidays. If you have an urgent medical problem that cannot wait until the start of our regular hours, please call 999-2222 to speak with one of our physicians. (*or* Please remain on the line. Our service operator will be with you shortly.)

Answering Services

Your answering service should be thought of as an extension of your office staff. When possible, meet with supervisors and operators personally. Your office policy manual together with careful written and verbal instructions should be given to service personnel. Documentation of calls should be discussed with supervisors, including the method of documentation used, length of time records are to be maintained, and how you are to gain access to these records. Although service operators should be discouraged from giving advice over the telephone, they constantly make triage decisions when deciding whether to hold calls or to page you. Their general instructions should be similar to those given to your receptionist in your office manual. Some operators report that having access to a telephone triage manual like this one is helpful when making these decisions. The best overall screening question for service operators to ask is simply "Is this call an emergency?" If the caller thinks the call is an emergency, the doctor on call should be paged.

Some communities have medical telephone answering services that

Common
Symptoms

Emergencies
and Traumas

Minor
Infections

Infectious
Diseases

Parenting
Concerns

Infant
Care

General
Principles

Common
Symptoms

Emergencies
and Traumas

Minor
Infections

Infectious
Diseases

Parenting
Concerns

Infant
Care

are maintained by supervised and trained professionals who will triage calls, offer advice, and refer patients to an agreed upon treatment site when the physician is off-call. These services can be very desirable, especially for solo practitioners with limited after-hours coverage, but they must be carefully evaluated for patient acceptance, suitability to practice style, and cost effectiveness. Parents' awareness that *their* doctor is available after-hours is often one of the most important factors in maintaining practice growth.

Answering service *performance* can be monitored by following up on complaints made by parents and patients and by occasionally calling for messages on the "patients'" phone line rather than using the "private" service line. Attention should be given to the length of time before calls are answered, the telephone manners and skill of the operator, and the number of times you are placed on hold.

Receptionist's Manual

A receptionist's manual should be prepared to include the topics listed below. The appendix of this book has pages that have been allocated for entry of this information if desired.

- *Travel instructions* to the office. (Use a format that can be faxed when necessary.)
- *Commonly used nonprescription medications* and their dose by age and weight.
- *Schedules* for immunization and physical examinations.
- *Triage instructions:* Follow the procedures outlined below.

Calls Requiring Immediate Attention
- Severe trauma, pain or parental anxiety.
- Calls from a physician or hospital about an ill patient.
SCREENING QUESTION. "The doctor is with a patient. Would you like me to interrupt her for you?"
- Calls that the parent believes are an emergency.
SCREENING QUESTION. "Is this problem an emergency?"

Calls Requiring Attention in the Near Future
- Acute illness (fever, upper respiratory tract infection, cough, vomiting, etc.).
- Calls from pharmacies concerning prescriptions.
- Minor trauma.

Routine (Nonemergent) Calls
- Infant care (feeding, bathing, diaper rash, etc.).

38

- Behavioral and school problems.
- Hospital or office business (billing, schedules, etc.).

Modifications to the priority schedule should be made to allow for personal and practice preferences. For example, the clinician may request immediate notification for all calls about ill children received 1 hour prior to office closing time.

- *Billing,* insurance, and other office business policies.
- *Telephone numbers* commonly used for pharmacies, suppliers, insurance companies, etc.
- *Consultants* commonly called by practice physicians: addresses and telephone numbers.
- *Professional and ancillary staff members:* addresses and primary and secondary telephone numbers.

Training Office Staff

Training sessions for office staff might include *sensitivity sessions* to discuss patient relations, telephone style, and office policy. *Role play* and *prepared scripts* can also be helpful for reviewing the most common medical conditions. These include fevers, coughs and colds, diarrhea and vomiting, and trauma. If *prepared manuals* like this one are to be used by the staff, the information in the manual should be carefully reviewed by the professional in charge, and reference copies should be made available at each of the commonly used telephone sites. The manual should be considered mandatory reading for all full- and part-time personnel, and documentation should be made after it has been read.

Teaching Parents Telephone Technique

When printed patient instructions are given, they should include the following topics. An example of patient instruction materials is included in the appendix on page 285.

- *Calling times.* Parents should call during office hours when possible. Emergency calls can be made at any time. Preferred calling times for nonurgent calls should be given.
- *Emergencies.* Callers should state "This is an emergency" to avoid confusion. Nonurgent calls should be identified in a similar manner.
- *Identification.* Callers should give the parent's name, the child's name, age, and sex, and the times and telephone numbers where they can be reached.

General Principles

Common Symptoms

Emergencies and Traumas

Minor Infections

Infectious Diseases

Parenting Concerns

Infant Care

39

General Principles

Common Symptoms

Emergencies and Traumas

Minor Infections

Infectious Diseases

Parenting Concerns

Infant Care

- *Symptoms.* The most important symptoms should be given first. Brevity is important, especially when talking with the receptionist or answering service operator. "Parent's intuition" is encouraged when describing the seriousness of a child's condition.
- *Background information.* The caller should be prepared to report the child's chronic or recurring illnesses, medicines or treatments currently being taken, recently received immunizations (shots), known allergies, medicines available in the home, and the telephone number of the local pharmacy.
- *Call-backs.* The caller should ask when the doctor or nurse is most likely to return the call. If there is no response within a reasonable period of time, the office should be called back to be certain that a misunderstanding has not occurred.
- *Record keeping.* Instructions received over the telephone should be written down for later reference.
- *Conclusion of the call.* Before hanging up, the caller should understand the most likely cause of the child's problem, which treatments, if any, are required, and under which circumstances to call back or make an appointment.
- *Travel.* If an office or hospital visit is required, the caller should have travel directions before leaving home and be certain to drive slowly and carefully. Alternate transportation should be requested for life-threatening emergencies or extreme anxiety.

Self-Evaluation

Constant self-evaluation is the key to maintaining good telephone skills. Poor telephone practices should be suspected when patients
- Frequently act angry or become argumentative with you or your staff.
- Do not seem reassured after advice has been offered.
- Complain that they are being told to come for "unnecessary" visits.
- Frequently have delayed diagnosis of serious illness despite earlier telephone contact.
- Have been told over the telephone to take medicines that interfered with diagnosis or treatment.
- Call back often to report trivial changes in a child's condition.
- Call back frequently to clarify instructions.
- Telephone during nights and weekends to ask questions or discuss matters that should more properly be discussed during regular office hours.

40

Patient Relations:
The Irate Parent

Despite our best intentions, parents sometimes become angry with practitioners, their ancillary staff, or their hospitals. It takes skill, time, and effort to defuse these situations. If left unattended, the problem of an irate parent escalates. When the problem is handled properly, you can make a new friend and feel good about yourself in the process. Angry parents need your help—not your anger in return.

Don't confuse anger directed *toward* you as meaning that a parent is angry *with* you. More commonly, he is angry at his situation. By offering your help, you also help yourself. One savvy communications specialist described what he calls the wonderful paradox: "I have more fun and enjoy more . . . success when I stop trying to get what I want, and start helping other people to get what they want." He also realized that "I quickly reduce my stress because I no longer try to get people to do what they don't want to do." When dealing with an unhappy parent, here are some tips that you might find helpful.

Use an Effective Introduction

The opening remarks set the tone for the rest of the conversation: "Hello Mr. Smith. My name is Dr. Raft. I am an associate here at Pediatric Associates. I can see that you are very upset today. What can I do to help you?" While this short introduction seems very simple, it contains several important elements:

- *Use of names.* By exchanging names you are personalizing the discussion. This is especially important in larger offices where the patient may not know all of the staff members.
- *Use of titles.* Give the parent your job description. It establishes your credentials and allows him to determine whether you are the right person to resolve this specific problem. Refer to the parent with a formal title (Mr., Miss, etc.) unless you have previously asked for permission or usually use his first name. This is polite and a sign that you respect his intelligence and opinion.

General
Principles

Common
Symptoms

Emergencies
and Traumas

Minor
Infections

Infectious
Diseases

Parenting
Concerns

Infant
Care

Attitude

It is not helpful to begin the call by sounding annoyed, disinterested, or angry. One angry person is enough! In most cases, the parent *wants* to have the problem resolved, even when this does not appear so initially. Despite his "attack," you must try to remain calm, interested, friendly, and helpful.

Redefine Winning

When you have a confrontation with a parent, you "win" only when he is happy with the final solution. This does *not* mean that you must win the argument. Your objective is not to beat the parent down; you simply want him to be satisfied with you and your service. Don't forget the golden rule of good patient relations: Treat your patients' families the way that *they* want to be treated.

Bond with the Caller

An angry parent is not your enemy. This is an opportunity to establish or improve on your relationship. When you say "I can see that you are very upset," you are making an obvious statement, but you are also letting the parent know that you are observant and sympathetic to his problem. If you said "Don't be upset," it would trivialize the complaint.

Offer Your Help

You are ready to give your help. Let the parent know it is all right to expect it.

Clarify the Problem

After a parent explains the problem, be sure that you understand it as he does. Some parents have great difficulty presenting facts concisely, and if they are agitated, essential elements may be left out of the discussion. It is helpful to summarize the complaint and repeat it back to the caller:

> I want to be sure that I understand your problem. At your appointment with Dr. Harris on Tuesday, she ordered laboratory work for your son. Blood was drawn and sent on Wednesday. The laborato-

ry mailed you a bill, but now our nurse says that there is no record of the test results. Is that correct?

Define Essential Elements

Before finding a reasonable solution to a problem, each element must be examined *separately*. In this case, there are two distinct issues: (1) The laboratory results are missing, and (2) if they cannot be found, the parent will be billed for services that were not received.

Request Supplemental Information

Ask additional questions that might expose an *obvious* mistake. In this example, the parent might have erred by going to the wrong laboratory, or he might not have given the correct doctor's name.

Assume the error is yours until proven otherwise. Do not make inquiries in a way that questions the parent's honesty or intelligence. The responses "Are you sure you went to the right laboratory?" and "Are you sure that you gave the technician Dr. Harris's name?" suggest that the error was the parent's fault. Less judgmental questions might be "What was the name of the laboratory that you went to?" and "Did you notice if the technician wrote Dr. Harris's name on the requisition slip?"

Review the Caller's Expectations

A solution that seems reasonable to you may not seem reasonable to the parent. If you are not sure which solution might make him happy, offer a choice: "If we can't locate the test results, I can make arrangements to have them repeated, or I can have the laboratory correct your bill. You might wish to speak with Dr. Harris before making your decision; I can have her call you tomorrow."

Be Sympathetic and Empathetic

The likelihood is that you would be angry if you were placed in this parent's position. Why not say so? Offering words of encouragement and understanding does not mean that you are being disloyal to those you work with. This is not a case of "us against them." A sympathetic attitude toward the parents reflects well on everyone at the office or clinic. You might say "I don't blame you for being angry. These tests were painful

Common Symptoms

Emergencies and Traumas

Minor Infections

Infectious Diseases

Parenting Concerns

Infant Care

General
Principles

Common
Symptoms

Emergencies
and Traumas

Minor
Infections

Infectious
Diseases

Parenting
Concerns

Infant
Care

for your son, and I know that you had to take a morning off from work. If this had happened to me, I would be angry too."

Offer an Apology

If the error was yours, say so. If it wasn't, apologize anyway. Most parents believe in the "captain of the ship" theory: If an accident occurs, the person in charge is held responsible—regardless of who committed the error. In this case, Pediatric Associates chose the laboratory. Even if the parent committed the error, he may hold you responsible if he believes that incomplete instructions were given. If you want to be thought of as being in charge, act as if you are. Accept this responsibility immediately without having it forced on you. Some appropriate responses include:

> I think I've found the problem. Our secretary misspelled your name on the requisition slip. I know she will feel badly when she finds out that you had so much difficulty.

> I think I've found the problem. The laboratory misspelled your name when it was entered into its computer. They were very apologetic. I'm sorry you were so inconvenienced.

> I think I've found the problem. You gave the laboratory your son's allergist's name instead of Dr. Harris's name, and the results were never mailed to our office. They are going to fax them to us. I feel badly that this happened, but I'll call you as soon as I receive them.

Follow up on the Problem

It is essential to learn whether the problem has been corrected as planned. A short phone call takes less time than having to explain why there has been another mix-up. You might also give the patient a phone number to call if the difficulty does not come to a successful conclusion. Most important, do not abandon the parent until you, personally, know that the matter has been resolved.

Other Considerations

Learn Preventive Techniques
It goes without saying that the best way to avoid problems is to prevent them. If you think that there is a high likelihood that a patient will be-

44

come upset about a particular situation, call to discuss it *before* she complains. If you learn that a message was inadvertently misplaced and a parent's call was never returned, apologize and explain why. If the patient was given a prescription in error, apologize while making the correction.

Establish Priorities
Complaints should receive first priority after medical emergencies. Parents with a grievance may have already been inconvenienced for hours, days, or weeks. The inconvenience to yourself and your present patients is the price that must sometimes be paid. Time lost can be minimized, however, when a sympathetic staff member who is less hurried can be assigned to call or speak with this parent until you are free and say: "Dr. Williams will be tied up with an emergency for the next hour or so. Is there something I can do to help you?"

Avoid Confrontational Responses
When you disagree with an angry parent, avoid saying so whenever possible. By openly disagreeing, you seem argumentative rather than accommodating. You can, however, respond by sounding sympathetic to his *interpretation* of the events but not necessarily to his *conclusions*. This sounds tricky and requires a little practice, but it is really quite simple. These responses are more likely to make a parent receptive to hearing your side of the story:

> I can understand why you might think that this was the case, but . . . .

> Many people feel exactly the same way you do, but there are some specific reasons why we have established this policy.

> We know that it looks as if our office is very inefficient when something like this happens, but . . . .

Avoid Patronizing Comments
"Don't be ridiculous" and "Don't be silly" are not good ways of opening a path toward good communication; they usually provoke frank hostility. An even angrier parent is likely to respond with "Don't tell me that I'm being ridiculous!"

Avoid Criticizing Other Staff Members
When a staff member has done or said something you believe to be inappropriate, discuss the matter with her in private. You can, however, offer the parent an apology that is not specifically critical of your workmate. An example might be "I'm sorry that you were upset by what our secretary said. Is there some way I can help you?"

General
Principles

Common
Symptoms

Emergencies
and Traumas

Minor
Infections

Infectious
Diseases

Parenting
Concerns

Infant
Care

Sometimes, together with an apology, it might be best to simply refer the parent back to the source of the problem: "I wish I could help you with this, but Ms. Robbins makes all of the office appointments. I think it would be best if she answers these questions for you. I will put her on the line. If she can't help you, please let me know."

Avoid Responding to a Complaint with a Complaint

A parent who says "I've been waiting for you to call back for a very long time" does not want to hear a complaint or a reprimand in response. Avoid saying "I haven't been sitting around doing nothing; I've been *very* busy" or "You wouldn't have had to wait so long if you had called me earlier in the day." Instead, try using statements that might make the delay an advantage to the parent: "I know that you have been waiting for a very long time, and I know that you're upset. I didn't call you back sooner because I didn't want to cut you short. If your problem is urgent, I can talk to you now. If it's not, let me call you back as soon as I finish seeing these sick patients and I am under less pressure."

Enjoy Your Reward

From the moment that a parent tells you about a problem, you become that parent's personal representative as a *problem-solving specialist.* Your reward should come from making him happy. Anyone can talk with parents who are friendly. Being able to satisfy unhappy parents shows that you have truly become skilled at doing your job properly.

Notes

General
Principles

Notes

Common
Symptoms

Emergencies
and Traumas

Minor
Infections

Infectious
Diseases

Parenting
Concerns

Infant
Care

Notes

Common
Symptoms

Emergencies
and Traumas

Minor
Infections

Infectious
Diseases

Parenting
Concerns

Infant
Care

Common Symptomatic Complaints

General Symptoms
Fever
Nonspecific Illness ("My Child
 Is Sick")
The Toxic Child

Respiratory Symptoms
Cough
Croup
Earache
Sore Throat
Upper Respiratory Infection
Wheezing

Gastrointestinal Symptoms
Abdominal Pain in Older
 Children
Constipation
Prolonged or Recurrent Infant
 Crying
Diarrhea
Vomiting

Other Symptoms
Headache
Pain on Urination
Skin Rashes

General
Principles

**Common
Symptoms**

Emergencies
and Traumas

Minor
Infections

Infectious
Diseases

Parenting
Concerns

Infant
Care

51

Fever

Screening Questions

Background
- Name, age, sex?
- Chronic illness?
- Current medications, treatments, or recent immunizations?

Severity
- How high is the fever?

Duration
- How long has fever been present?

Other Symptoms
- Have you noticed any other symptoms such as runny nose, cough, vomiting, diarrhea, or rash?

Pain
- Does your child seem to have discomfort or complain of pain in the ears, throat, stomach, or head?

General Appearance
- Does your child seem especially sick?

Examine Immediately If

- The child appears toxic.
- There is extreme parental anxiety.
- Temperature is greater than 105°F (40.6°C) after fever-lowering medication has been given.
- There is a rash that looks like bruising or bleeding under the skin.
- Temperature is greater than 101°F (38.4°C) when the child is less than 3 months old.

Jeffrey L. Brown: *Pediatric Telephone Medicine: Principles, Triage, and Advice,* Second Edition. Copyright © 1994 J. B. Lippincott Company

General
Principles

Common
Symptoms

Emergencies
and Traumas

Minor
Infections

Infectious
Diseases

Parenting
Concerns

Infant
Care

Examine in the Near Future If

- There is persistent temperature greater than 101°F (38.8°C) for longer than 24 hours.
- There is intermittent temperature greater than 101°F (38.8°C) for more than 3 days.
- There are other significant associated symptoms.

See Related Sections

The toxic child (p. 61), convulsions (p. 163).

Treatment

- *Reassurance.* Children often have temperature greater than 102°F (38.8°C) associated with minor illnesses, including upper respiratory tract infections.
- *Medication.* An aspirin substitute may be prescribed for symptom relief. If the child feels hot to the touch 20 minutes after administration of medicine, the parent may wish to take the child's temperature again.

  Acetaminophen is usually given at 15 mg/kg and repeatedly every 4 hours as needed; ibuprofen is usually given at 10 mg/kg and repeatedly every 6 hours as needed. When adjusted for dose, these medicines have similar efficacy.
- *Sponging.* If the child feels uncomfortable and the rectal temperature is greater than 104°F (40°C) after fever-reducing medicines have been given, he should be placed in a partially filled tub of lukewarm water for 10 to 20 minutes. Alcohol should not be added to the bathwater or applied to the child's skin.
- *Clothing.* The child should be dressed in loose-fitting, lightweight cotton clothing to absorb perspiration. If the child feels cold or has actual chills, he may be covered briefly with a lightweight blanket for comfort. Room temperature should be kept toward the cool side; an air conditioner is helpful during summer months.
- *Diet.* A light diet consisting of soft, bland foods should be offered. Calorie-containing liquids (not diet soda or plain water) can be offered if solids are refused.
- *Examination.* When the child has high fever for a prolonged period of time, his body should be examined regularly for the appearance of a rash. If a rash develops that has the appearance of bruising or bleeding under the skin, it should be reported immediately.

54

CLINICAL TIP. Most antipyretics are dosed so that 1 adult tablet is the equivalent of 2 teaspoonfuls, 2 junior tablets, 4 infant droppers, or 4 baby tablets. A typical 12-year-old gets the equivalent of 2 adult tablets, a 6-year-old 1 adult tablet (2 teaspoonfuls of elixir), an 18-month-old 1 teaspoonful of elixir, and a 3-month-old 1 baby dropperful. When dosages are adjusted, patients will usually receive equal volumes of the same dose form of acetaminophen and ibuprofen. Become familiar with alternate dose forms such as sprinkles and suppositories. These can be very helpful for children who are oppositional or vomiting.

Approximate doses of commonly used antipyretics are as follows:

Acetaminophen 80 mg/0.8 ml dropper: 1 dropper for each 12 lb

Acetaminophen 80 mg baby tablets: 1 tablet for each 12 lb

Acetaminophen syrup 160 mg/tsp: 1 teaspoon for each 25 lb

Acetaminophen 160 mg junior chew tabs: 1 tablet for each 25 lb

Acetaminophen 300 mg adult tablet: 1 tablet for each 50 lb

Ibuprofen syrup 100 mg/tsp: 1 teaspoon for each 25 lb

Ibuprofen adult 200 mg/tablet: 1 tablet for each 50 lb

Parent Call-back Is Needed for

- Persistent, changing, worsening, anxiety-provoking, or specific symptoms.

Discussion

Fever can be the most anxiety-provoking of symptoms for parents. *Fever phobias* continue to be fueled by professionals, friends, relatives, and others who believe that high fever is a cause of brain damage. Excluding heat stroke, there is virtually no evidence to suggest that this is true, and many experts believe that fever has a beneficial effect in helping body defenses to fight infection. Febrile convulsions have not been shown to be associated with brain damage and are not more likely than fever alone to be associated with meningitis. Good teaching opportunities include times

Emergencies
and Traumas

Minor
Infections

Infectious
Diseases

Parenting
Concerns

Infant
Care

General
Principles

Common
Symptoms

Emergencies
and Traumas

Minor
Infections

Infectious
Diseases

Parenting
Concerns

Infant
Care

when parents are given instructions about febrile illness or possible vaccine reactions. Both in-person and telephone discussions about fever should cover the following elements.

- The general appearance of the child is often a better guide to the severity of illness than the degree of the fever. Parents should be more concerned about an ill-appearing child with low-grade fever than one with high fever who appears alert and well. Children with roseola commonly have temperatures of 104°F (40°C) and 105°F (40.6°C) for 2 or 3 days but don't appear especially sick.
- Younger children tend to run higher fevers than older children and adults.
- Fever tends to be higher at night than during the daytime.
- Fever is a normal body response to infection and other conditions and probably helps body defenses to work better.
- High fevers can seem frightening, but parents should remember that they do not cause brain damage except when they are associated with heat stroke.
- Fever is treated more to relieve discomfort than to lower temperature. When a febrile child is alert and appears well, no treatment is necessary. When the child acts uncomfortable, fever reducers can help to make her feel better.
- In most cases, febrile children do not have to be awakened from sleep to be given fever-reducers. But if they do wake up and feel ill, medicine may be useful to help them return to sleep.
- *Optional:* A small percentage of children will develop convulsions when they have fever. In most cases, these convulsions will stop after a few minutes without treatment. A child with a fever convulsion usually requires evaluation, but the convulsions themselves do not cause brain or neurological damage.

Sponging should only be used if temperature is high and the child seems uncomfortable after fever-lowering medicines have been given. Bathwater should feel just comfortable to the hand. Placing the child in water that is too cool, especially without first lowering the child's "brain thermostat" with acetaminophen or ibuprofen, may cause shivering and an initial increase in temperature. Alcohol should not be used either in the bathwater or on the skin. The benefit of alcohol evaporation is minimal, and when alcohol is used in an underventilated room, inhaled vapor can lead to alcohol intoxication, low blood sugar, and seizures.

To avoid unnecessary call-backs, an authoritative manner should be used when discussing fever. Without good technique, one will regularly be examining the well-appearing but febrile children of fever-phobic parents at 3:00 A.M.; these children will have more energy than the doctor, the parents, or the bleary-eyed emergency room staff.

Infants less than 3 months old require earlier evaluation than older children. It is more difficult to assess degree of illness over the phone, and there is a greater likelihood for missing serious illness. Many physicians believe that all febrile babies should be examined immediately. Certainly, any infant with a rectal temperature greater than 101°F (38.4°C) who is feeding poorly, irritable, or has other symptoms should be examined as quickly as is practical. However, when a known reliable parent reports that a febrile infant looks well, is feeding and acting normally, and has no other significant symptoms, a repeat rectal temperature taken 3 or 4 hours later might be requested before an immediate examination is suggested. If the baby is not seen immediately, it is imperative to maintain close telephone contact and to keep written records of the baby's progress.

Screening questions for febrile children are purposefully broad. Most children with fever have some degree of irritability, lethargy, and loss of appetite. *Stiff neck* was not included as a screening question because this sign or symptom can be difficult to evaluate even when a child is examined in-person. Febrile children frequently complain of headache, muscle aches (especially at the flank and back of the neck), and joint pains. If a child can place his chin on his chest with ease, nuchal rigidity is unlikely. But many older febrile children complain of some discomfort when asked to flex their necks; younger children often refuse; and most parents are not skilled at determining when neck stiffness is involuntary. Once the question has been asked, interpreting the answer is often difficult, and the anxiety and uncertainty that follow can be more troublesome to both parents and clinicians than the information gained. Febrile children with tender submandibular nodes or earache sometimes complain of stiff neck. Those without fever may have torticollis after awakening from an uncomfortable sleeping position, or they may have experienced minor trauma causing muscle strain.

When there is a *rash* that looks like bruising or bleeding under the skin, it may reflect early signs of meningococcemia, *Haemophilus influenzae* sepsis, or other serious infections that require immediate evaluation. One advantage of sponging children with high fever is that the parent can visualize the child's entire body when he is placed in the tub. If sponging is not being used, repeat visual inspection at regular intervals is recommended.

History taking should include questions about recent *immunizations* as well as other symptoms. Diphtheria, pertussis, tetanus (DPT) vaccine is a common cause of fever in young infants, and measles vaccine can cause a febrile reaction 5 to 10 days later. However, the history of a recent immunization and the presence of fever do not always mean that there is a causal relationship. Degree of illness must still be assessed when deciding whether an examination is needed even when an immunization reaction is the most likely cause.

Avoid discussing *fever convulsions* unless you have been specifically

General Principles

Common Symptoms

Emergencies and Traumas

Minor Infections

Infectious Diseases

Parenting Concerns

Infant Care

General
Principles

Common
Symptoms

Emergencies
and Traumas

Minor
Infections

Infectious
Diseases

Parenting
Concerns

Infant
Care

asked about them. The discussion may provoke more anxiety than it relieves. It sometimes helps to remind parents that the only significant risk from fever convulsions is not from the convulsion itself but from a possible automobile accident when the parent races to the emergency room.

Some parents express apprehension about *taking the child outdoors* when going to the office, clinic, or emergency room for an examination. Remind them that cool baths are used to treat fever and air conditioners are used for febrile symptoms during summer months, so taking the child outside should not be a problem. In fact, the trip outside frequently lowers rather than raises the temperature.

Only *rectal thermometers* are truly accurate, with ear probes and axillary temperatures taken with an oral thermometer second bests. Oral temperatures should not be used for young children.

A *waiting time* commensurate with the child's appearance and symptom complex may be helpful for increasing the *effective yield* of appropriate examinations. Children seen immediately after the onset of fever are more likely to have spontaneous resolution of symptoms and a paucity of findings at examination than those examined after 24 hours of elevated temperature. This strategy has the additional benefit of improving patient flow through a busy office or clinic and reinforces the idea that fever alone is not a serious symptom that requires immediate attention or treatment.

Nonspecific Illness ("My Child Is Sick")

Screening Questions

Background
- Name, age, sex?
- Chronic illness?
- Current medications, treatments, or recent immunizations?

Fever
- If fever is present, how high is it and when did it begin?

Respiratory Symptoms
- Does your child have a runny nose, cough, or difficulty breathing?

Gastrointestinal Symptoms
- Does your child have cramps, vomiting, or diarrhea?

Skin
- Does your child have a rash?

Others Symptoms
- Are there any other symptoms that you are worried about?

General Appearance
- Does the child look especially sick?
- Do you feel frightened about the way your child looks?

Examination

- Depends on the specific illness.

See Related Sections

The toxic child (p. 61).

Jeffrey L. Brown: *Pediatric Telephone Medicine: Principles, Triage, and Advice,*
Second Edition. Copyright © 1994 J. B. Lippincott Company

General
Principles

Common
Symptoms

Emergencies
and Traumas

Minor
Infections

Infectious
Diseases

Parenting
Concerns

Infant
Care

Treatment

- Depends on the specific illness.

Parent Call-back Is Needed For

- Persistent, changing, worsening, anxiety-provoking, or specific symptoms.

Discussion

Parents may describe their child's illness in nonspecific terms, saying "My child is sick" when they are feeling anxious, when they have poor verbal skills, or when they are not really calling for advice but need the reassurance of just "checking in." Also a runny nose without other symptoms assumes more importance when it is presented as a diagnostic challenge. If the parent simply said "My child has a cold," the call might sound more trivial.

The great majority of these calls are made for routine rather than serious illness, and clustering questions by symptom-groups together with a rapid assessment of general condition can be accomplished quickly: "Does your child have a fever?"

"No."

"Does he have a cough, cold, sore throat, or runny nose?"

"No."

"Does he have a stomachache, vomiting, or diarrhea?

"No."

"Does he have a rash, or are there any specific symptoms that you are concerned about?"

Once specific symptoms are given, they must be evaluated individually; when the complaint sounds trivial, don't forget to inquire about hidden agendas. (See p. 12.)

The Toxic Child

Screening Questions

Background
- Name, age, sex?
- Chronic illness?
- Current medications, treatments, or recent immunizations?

General Appearance
- Does your child look sicker than usual with most illnesses?
- Do you feel especially frightened by the way he looks?
- Does he look sick as he would from a cold, or does he look much sicker than that?
- What has your child been doing during the past few hours?
- All children are more sleepy than usual when they become ill, but how does your child appear when he is up and around?

Breathing
- Is his breathing strained, or does he have to work hard to move air in and out?
- Is his breathing shallow and rapid?
- Is his chest heaving when he breathes?
- Does he make a grunting noise or moan with each breath?

Skin
- Is his skin cold and clammy?
- Is his skin gray, bluish, or dusky?
- Does he have a rash that looks like bleeding or bruising under the skin?

Neurological Assessment for Infants Less than 8 Weeks Old

- Is he very lethargic and difficult to arouse?
- Does his body seem limp?
- Has he been feeding badly for two or more consecutive feedings?

Jeffrey L. Brown: *Pediatric Telephone Medicine: Principles, Triage, and Advice,*
Second Edition. Copyright © 1994 J. B. Lippincott Company

General
Principles

Common
Symptoms

Emergencies
and Traumas

Minor
Infections

Infectious
Diseases

Parenting
Concerns

Infant
Care

- Is his crying weak or feeble?
- Has he been extremely irritable for more than 4 hours and cannot be calmed when he is held, rocked, or fed?

Neurological Assessment for Older Children

- Is he extremely lethargic and difficult to arouse?
- Does his body seem limp?
- If more than 3 months old, does he seem so sick that he can't make eye contact with you and seem to be staring off into space?
- Does he show signs of confused or disoriented thinking?

Examine Immediately If

- You believe the child to be toxic. (See discussion.)

Examine in the Near Future If

- The child appears sicker than usual for "routine" illnesses.

Discussion

The term "looking toxic" suggests that the observer has a subjective feeling that this child appears *gravely ill*. No single finding can convey this feeling; it is based on past experience and intuition as well as observation. Since only the caretaker can make observations of the child's appearance during telephone contacts, one must rely on descriptive language to make this assessment. Questions should be directive but not leading and should employ terminology appropriate to the caretaker's ethnicity, personality, and educational level.

A "yes" answer to any of the screening questions listed above should signal interest but not necessarily alarm; most positive responses can also be associated with nonserious illness: A child who is vomiting or who has just struck his head during a fall may transiently appear pale, sweaty, and have rapid, shallow breathing; one awakened from deep sleep may initially appear disoriented or confused; and babies with colic may have prolonged periods of inconsolable crying. The more "yes" answers received to these screening questions and the longer the duration of symptoms, the more concerned the practitioner should become.

It is not always time-effective and frequently not necessary to ask more than one or two questions to assess toxicity, but it is necessary to get an overview of the child's overall condition. "Does your child look much sicker than when she gets a routine illness like a cold or stomach virus?" is a simple screen to see whether a more detailed history is necessary. When a firm conclusion cannot be reached about the child's general appearance, the question "Do you feel frightened about the way your child looks?" allows the caretaker to collate subjective feelings that cannot otherwise be put into words. Affirmative responses that can't be qualified with a simple explanation should prompt in-person evaluation as soon as it is practical.

General
Principles

Common
Symptoms

Emergencies
and Traumas

Minor
Infections

Infectious
Diseases

Parenting
Concerns

Infant
Care

Cough

Screening Questions

Background
- Name, age, sex?
- Chronic illness?
- Current medications and treatments?

Duration
- How long have symptoms been present?

Fever
- If there is fever, how high is it and how long has it been present?

Timing
- Is the cough present all day or only at night and on awakening?

Character
- Is the cough loose, tight and staccato (multiple dry brief coughs), or barking (like a seal or dog)?

Other Symptoms
- Does the child have hoarseness, a runny nose, or signs of allergy (itchy eyes and nose)?

Breathing Difficulty
- Does the child have wheezing?
- Does the child have labored breathing?
- Is the child straining to get air in and out, or is his chest heaving when he breathes?

Sputum Characteristics (over 12 years old)
- If the child spits out sputum (phlegm) after coughing, does it look green or yellow like pus?

General Appearance
- Does the child look especially sick?

General
Principles

Common
Symptoms

Emergencies
and Traumas

Minor
Infections

Infectious
Diseases

Parenting
Concerns

Infant
Care

Examine Immediately If

- The child appears toxic.
- There is wheezing or labored breathing that has lasted longer than 30 minutes that has not responded to symptomatic treatment.
- The child is less than 3 months old and has rapid breathing, wheezing, or constant cough (every 5 to 10 minutes).
- There is extreme parental anxiety.

Examine in the Near Future If

- Temperature is greater than 101°F (38.4°C) for longer than 24 hours.
- Coughing persists all day.
- The cough has a staccato or croupy (barking) quality.
- Wheezing lasts longer than 24 hours even with minimal breathing difficulty.
- An infant less than 3 months old has a persistent cough.
- Symptoms have lasted longer than 10 days.

See Related Sections

The toxic child (p. 61), upper respiratory infection (p. 81), wheezing (p. 85), croup (p. 69), fever (p. 53), pertussis (p. 231).

Treatment

- Consider decongestant nose drops for upper respiratory tract symptoms when children are older than 6 months or oral decongestants when children are older than 5 years.
- Raise the head-end of the child's bed using a rolled blanket under the mattress or by placing books under the legs of the bed.
- Use a vaporizer or inhaled steam if the cough is associated with mouth breathing or with croup.
- Administer cough suppressants at night if the child's coughing prevents sleep.
- Bronchodilators may be given to the older child with persistent wheezing or to a child with suspected bronchospasm.
- Antihistamines may be of value for the child with allergic symptoms.

Parent Call-Back Is Needed for

- Persistent, changing, worsening, anxiety-provoking, or specific symptoms as outlined above.

Discussion

Coughing associated with *upper respiratory tract infections* and *allergy* is usually loose and worsens when the child is in the sleeping position. *Lower respiratory infections* (bronchitis and pneumonia) and bronchospasm are more commonly associated with a persistent, short, staccato cough that is worse in prone or supine position; this cough is present all day, may be worse at night, and may be precipitated by exercise. True wheezing and fever are also more likely to represent lower airway disease. Children younger than 3 months old who have a constant cough are presumed to have *pneumonia* and should be examined as soon as practical. Known asthmatics and others suspected of having *bronchospasm* should be treated as outlined in the section on wheezing.

Coughing from *pertussis* (whooping cough) has a characteristic inhaled "whooping" sound after a bout of coughing. The child may have a history of recent severe rhinitis, appear ill, have color change associated with coughing, and vomit following a coughing spasm. Immunized adults and older children may have modified symptoms of whooping cough that suggest bronchitis. Despite immunization, this illness is still seen in many communities.

A barking cough occurring late at night that is associated with noisy breathing and hoarse voice is suggestive of *croup*. Steam is the primary treatment, although exposure to cold air may also bring relief. Steroids and inhaled racemic epinephrine are commonly prescribed for symptoms that don't resolve after home treatment.

Decongestant treatment of *upper respiratory symptoms* will usually provide relief from coughing. *Cough suppressants* should be used only when discomfort is severe or when older children have frequent disruption of sleep. Although daytime use of cough suppressants may make the child sound better, they can interfere with the child's ability to cough up secretions. Nonprescription cough suppressants appear to have minimal efficacy.

General
Principles

Common
Symptoms

Emergencies
and Traumas

Minor
Infections

Infectious
Diseases

Parenting
Concerns

Infant
Care

Croup (Laryngotracheal Bronchitis, Barking Cough)

Screening Questions

Background
- Name, age, sex?
- Chronic illness?
- Current medications and treatments?

Duration
- How long have symptoms been present?

Difficulty Breathing
- Does the child have to strain, "pull," or work hard to move air in and out?
- Does the child have wheezing when breathing in and breathing out or only when breathing out?

Fever
- If fever is present, how high is it and how long has it been present?

Color
- Does the child's color appear dusky or bluish, especially around the lips or at the fingertips?

Drooling
- Is saliva drooling from the child's mouth?
- Does the child sit up and lean forward to breathe more easily?

Other Symptoms
- Does the child have a cold, hoarseness, or other signs of illness?

General Appearance
- Does the child look especially sick?

Examine Immediately If

- The child appears toxic.
- There is no response to steam after 15 to 20 minutes.
- The child has extreme difficulty breathing, cyanosis, drooling, or requires a sitting and leaning-forward position to breathe more easily.
- There is extreme parental anxiety.

Examine in the Near Future If

- The croupy cough is present during the daytime.
- The child is younger than 1 year or older than 7 years.
- Symptoms persist for longer than 8 hours.

See Related Sections

The toxic child (p. 61), fever (p. 53), upper respiratory infection (p. 81), cough (p. 65), wheezing (p. 85).

Treatment

- Expose the child to steam by running hot water in the bathroom with the doors and windows closed for approximately 15 to 20 minutes. Later, place the child in a bed or a crib with a vaporizer aimed toward the head-end of the child's bed. She should then be checked at frequent intervals to be certain that labored breathing does not return.
- Decongestants may be given if rhinitis is present.
- Oral steroids may be indicated for children who have had recurrent episodes of croup.
- Treatment failures sometimes respond when a properly dressed child is placed sitting near an open window. When children are taken outside to be evaluated at a medical facility, they frequently show improvement by the time of arrival.

Parent Call-back Is Needed For

- Persistent, changing, worsening, anxiety-provoking, or specific symptoms as outlined above.

Discussion

Epiglottitis and *bacterial croup* are often associated with drooling, high fever, and leaning forward to improve breathing. These conditions may be life-threatening and, when suspected, should be evaluated immediately. *Viral croup* is often associated with a concurrent upper respiratory tract infection. *Spasmodic croup* tends to be recurrent and has sudden onset without antecedent symptoms; it is most often associated with change of seasons (in early winter and early spring).

All variations of croup cause extreme anxiety for both the child and the parent when they are awakened in the middle of the night by the foghorn sound of a barking cough. Parents who have not previously experienced this condition can be understandably reluctant to believe that steam is the mainstay of treatment. The child should be evaluated 15 to 20 minutes after breathing steam at a time when there is no crying and no coughing. If there is no difficulty breathing at rest, she can be returned to bed even when the barking cough or noisy breathing has continued. If symptoms are absent by morning, parents can use a bedside vaporizer during the next two to three nights because of the possibility of recurrence.

Some children also improve after vomiting or after being taken out into the cold night air. Practiced parents sometimes report that when their children fail to respond to steam, they roll down the car windows and drive around the block a few times with the child before going to the emergency room. Home administration of oral corticosteroids is sometimes recommended when the diagnosis is not in doubt.

Earache (Otitis)

Screening Questions

Background
- Name, age, sex?
- Chronic illness?
- Current medications and treatments?

Duration
- How long have symptoms been present?

Fever
- If there is fever, how high is it and how long has it been present?

Pain
- Is the pain especially severe, and is it affected by moving the outer ear?

Discharge
- Is fluid draining from the ear?

Other Symptoms
- Does the child have a runny nose or sore throat?

General Condition
- Does the child look especially sick?

Examine Immediately If

- The child appears toxic.

Examine in the Near Future If

- Ear pain lasts longer than 1 hour, even when symptoms disappear spontaneously.

- Temperature is greater than 101°F (38.4°C) for more than 1 day.
- Ear discharge is present.

See Related Sections

The toxic child (p. 61), swimmer's ear (p. 191), upper respiratory infection (p. 81), fever (p. 53).

Treatment

- Oral analgesics such as acetaminophen.
- Anesthetic ear drops if no ear discharge is present.
- Oral decongestants if rhinitis is present.
- Heat applied to the outer ear.
- Upright positioning of the patient.
- Much reassurance to both the parent and the patient.

Treatment for Otitis Externa (Swimmer's Ear)

When there are no systemic symptoms and pain is present only with manipulation of the outer ear:
- Heat applied to the outer ear.
- Ear drops containing antibiotics, acetic acid, steroids or combinations of these.
- Avoidance of water in the ear.

Parent Call-back Is Needed for

- Persistent, changing, worsening, anxiety-provoking, or specific symptoms as outlined above.

Discussion

Children with otitis media frequently have had a cold for a few days, lie down for sleep, awaken a few hours later with severe ear pain, which improves several hours later with or without treatment. The pain may be described as a dull ache but may be of such intensity that they literally scream for hours in distress.

The *diagnosis* of otitis media is very likely when an older febrile child has an earache, or when a younger child with a recent history of otitis media is febrile and pulling at her ears. *Other conditions* that may be confused with otitis media include dental abscess, early mumps, temperomandibular joint (TMJ) pain, and referred pain from pharyngitis or tonsillitis. Children less than 2 years old with acute otitis media may have fever without other signs or crying without localization of pain. *Ear discharge,* even with minor symptoms, should always be investigated. An inflamed tympanic membrane may melt wax in the ear canal, or pus may be draining through a perforated ear drum.

Symptomatic relief can be obtained by placing the child in an upright position; lying flat almost always makes pain worse. Heat should be applied to the outer ear. Analgesics and decongestants can be given immediately. Cough preparations containing decongestants and codeine are especially useful and when given together with acetaminophen will usually provide significant relief within 20 minutes. Analgesic ear drops may be helpful and have the psychological advantage of applying medicine to the place that hurts.

Advise parents that there is usually *spontaneous resolution* of ear pain after 4 to 8 hours, making an emergency trip to the hospital or pharmacy unnecessary. Also remind them of the *need for examination* even after the child has become asymptomatic.

Children may resume normal *activity* when they are symptom-free. Bathing, including hair washing and swimming, is allowed since the infection is on the inner side of the tympanic membrane. Activities affecting ear pressure, such as underwater diving and commercial air flights, should be avoided when possible.

Swimmer's ear (otitis externa) is more common during summer months and is suggested if ear pain becomes more intense when the outer ear is manipulated, especially when pressure is applied to the buttonlike structure (the tragus) in front of the ear. Since external otitis is essentially a skin irritation within the ear canal, systemic symptoms are not usually present.

General
Principles

Common
Symptoms

Emergencies
and Traumas

Minor
Infections

Infectious
Diseases

Parenting
Concerns

Infant
Care

Sore Throat (Pharyngitis)

General Principles

Common Symptoms

Emergencies and Traumas

Minor Infections

Infectious Diseases

Parenting Concerns

Infant Care

Screening Questions

Background
- Name, age, sex?
- Chronic illness?
- Current medications and treatments?

Duration
- How long have symptoms been present?

Fever
- Does the child have fever?
- If so, how high is it, and how long has it been present?

Other Symptoms
- Does the child have a runny nose, cough, hoarseness (laryngitis), or tender swollen glands in the neck?
- If a rash is present, does it look like a sunburn or like bruising or bleeding under the skin?

Breathing
- Does the child have difficulty breathing or have drooling from the mouth?

Strep Exposure
- Was there recent exposure to streptococcal infection?

General Appearance
- Does the child look especially sick?

Examine Immediately If

- The child appears toxic.
- There is difficulty breathing or drooling from the mouth.
- A rash is present that looks like bruising or bleeding under the skin.

Jeffrey L. Brown: *Pediatric Telephone Medicine: Principles, Triage, and Advice,* Second Edition. Copyright © 1994 J. B. Lippincott Company

General Principles

Common Symptoms

Emergencies and Traumas

Minor Infections

Infectious Diseases

Parenting Concerns

Infant Care

Examine in the Near Future If

- Temperature is greater than 101°F (38.4°C) for more than 24 hours.
- Tender swelling is present in the neck.
- The child has a rash that suggests a sunburn.
- There has been recent exposure to streptococcal infection.
- There is a known high prevalence of streptococcal infection in the community.
- Throat pain is severe and is present all through the day.
- Throat pain has lasted longer than 3 days.

See Related Sections

The toxic child (p. 61), fever (p. 53), upper respiratory infection (p. 81), and scarlatina (p. 229).

Treatment

- Acetaminophen for symptomatic relief of fever and pain.
- Throat lozenges, sucking candy, or honey to relieve throat pain.

Parent Call-back Is Needed for

- Persistent, changing, worsening, anxiety-provoking, or specific symptoms as outlined above.

Discussion

Only a positive throat culture or rapid strep test can confirm the diagnosis of streptococcal pharyngitis. In most cases, deferring treatment 24 to 48 hours will not significantly increase the likelihood of developing the infrequent heart and kidney complications associated with group A streptococcal infections. The advantages of early treatment may lie in the prevention of serious illness for exposed siblings and earlier resolution of acute symptoms for infected children.

When there has been recent exposure to group A streptococcal infection or it is a *prevalent community illness,* an early examination should be performed even when minimal symptoms are present. *High temperature,* tender adenopathy, and severe pharyngeal pain are more commonly associated with streptococcal than viral pharyngitis. *Early morning pain* is more likely to be associated with mouth breathing during sleep, with subsequent drying of the mucous membranes. *All-day pain* is more likely to be from significant pharyngeal infection. *Laryngitis* and *runny nose* suggest viral infection but should be evaluated when symptoms persist or when other risk factors are present. *Signs of toxicity,* especially when accompanied by a rash, difficulty breathing, or drooling, should prompt early examination because of the possibility of *scarlatina* or *peritonsillar abscess.* A scarlatiniform rash might be described as a generalized sunburn that is worse under the arms and in the groin. When the child with a sore throat and fever develops a rash that looks like *bruising* or bleeding under the skin, it is suggestive of meningococcemia, *Haemophilus* influenza, or another form of bacterial sepsis, and immediate examination is therefore necessary.

Symptomatic treatment of minor throat pain with analgesics, topical anesthetics, or medicines that coat the throat are helpful to relieve discomfort. Be wary of suggesting use of throat lozenges and sucking candy for young children who may choke on them. Whenever possible, avoid prescribing antibiotics over the telephone. Many children with streptococcal sore throats will remain culture-positive after one or two doses of antibiotics, but it is preferred to avoid prescribing medicine until after the culture has been taken. An exception might be for the symptomatic sibling of a child with proven strep throat who cannot be brought to the office or clinic for evaluation. When pain occurs in association with mouth breathing, especially during winter months, humidification of air may help to soothe dry mucous membranes.

General Principles

Common Symptoms

Emergencies and Traumas

Minor Infections

Infectious Diseases

Parenting Concerns

Infant Care

General
Principles

Common
Symptoms

Emergencies
and Traumas

Minor
Infections

Infectious
Diseases

Parenting
Concerns

Infant
Care

Upper Respiratory Infection (URI, Rhinitis, Cold)

Screening Questions

Background
- Name, age, sex?
- Chronic illness?
- Current medications and treatments or recent immunizations?

Duration
- How long have symptoms been present?

Fever
- If fever is present, how high is it and when did it begin?

Nasal Discharge
- Is nasal discharge clear or does it look thick, yellow, or green like pus?
- If it looks like pus, is it intermittent or constant?

Cough
- If cough is present, does it occur all day or only nights and mornings?

Pain
- Does the child complain of throat or ear pain?

General Appearance
- Does the child look especially sick?

Examine Immediately If

- The child appears toxic.

Jeffrey L. Brown: *Pediatric Telephone Medicine: Principles, Triage, and Advice,*
Second Edition. Copyright © 1994 J. B. Lippincott Company

General
Principles

Common
Symptoms

Emergencies
and Traumas

Minor
Infections

Infectious
Diseases

Parenting
Concerns

Infant
Care

Examine in the Near Future If

- Upper respiratory symptoms have lasted longer than 10 days.
- Temperature has been persistently higher than 101°F (38.4°C) for longer than 24 hours.
- Purulent rhinitis or sore throat has been present for more than 3 days.
- Persistent cough is associated with wheezing, as an all-day symptom, or has a staccato quality.

See Related Sections

The toxic child (p. 61) fever (p. 53), pharyngitis (p. 77), cough (p. 65).

Treatment for Infants Less than 6 Months Old

- Normal saline solution may be used as nose drops before feedings and at bedtime.
- Nasal aspirator can be helpful for active rhinitis.
- Vaporizer for mouth breathing in dry-heated room.
- Prop up the head-end of the crib mattress.

Treatment for Children Older than 6 Months

- Oral decongestant for children older than 6 years and if found to be effective for children under age 6.
- Humidifier for mouth breathing in a dry room.
- Cough suppressant for children over 3 years of age at night if necessary.
- Antihistamine if allergic symptoms are suspected.

Parent Call-back Is Needed for

- Persistent, changing, worsening, anxiety-provoking, or specific symptoms as outlined above.

Discussion

During winter months clinicians spend so much time discussing cold symptoms that they can become desensitized to parental concerns and frustration. Two colds in sequence lasting 10 days each cause 3 weeks of illness. Parents trapped in the house with sick children must cope with fever, fretful sleeping patterns, poor eating, fights about taking medicine, arranging for baby-sitters, missed school and work, missed play dates and activities, and cranky behavior. Telephone calls about colds reflect all of these concerns, in addition to those caused by the illusion of serious illness when the child has audible rhonchi, coughing, and fever.

Examination is recommended when children have *temperature* greater than 101°F (38.4°C) for longer than 24 hours to evaluate the possibility of secondary infection. Parents should be told that *intermittent fever* commonly occurs anytime during the 7- to 10-day course of illness. When temperature is less than 101°F (38.4°C) it can usually be ignored in the absence of other significant symptoms.

Nasal discharge can be intermittently purulent during a cold, but persistence of thick green or yellow mucus is commonly associated with secondary infection such as sinusitis or otitis.

Coughing in the supine position is expected because of postnasal drip. However, a cough persisting throughout the day may be the result of bronchial irritation. Other signs of bronchial irritation include wheezing and a frequent, short dry coughing pattern.

Use of oral *decongestants* for children younger than 6 years old is controversial. Despite little evidence confirming efficacy, decongestants have remained very popular with parents because of their need "to do something" when their children are sick with a cold. These medicines frequently cause irritability and sleeplessness that can be mistaken for worsening signs of illness. Parents who prefer to give them anyway can be told to continue treatment if there are no obvious side effects and there seems to be significant improvement; the medication should be stopped if it is ineffective. Symptom-relieving medicines should be given when symptoms bother the child, not when they bother the parent. If a child's nighttime cough wakes the parent but not the child, no medicine is necessary.

Administration of *nose drops,* especially nonprescription normal saline solution, is a benign treatment for rhinitis in infants. Drops should be used prior to feedings and sleep to facilitate sucking and resting behaviors. Decongestant nose drops are very helpful and effective for children older than 6 months. They should only be used for consecutive periods of 5 days or less to avoid rebound worsening of rhinitis when they are discontinued.

Vaporizers and *humidifiers* have more psychological than practical

General Principles

Common Symptoms

Emergencies and Traumas

Minor Infections

Infectious Diseases

Parenting Concerns

Infant Care

benefit. They are useful, however, to keep the oropharynx moist when mouth breathing dry heated air during winter months, but mold contamination almost always occurs, offsetting potential benefit. Adding medication to the vaporoizer water should be discouraged since it may induce bronchospasm. Cool mist may be preferred to hot steam because of safety factors. Placing a large pot of water in the room may be an effective substitute for vaporizers and humidifiers and avoids the hazard of mold contamination.

Sore throat that is present on awakening but improves as the day progresses is commonly caused by dryness from mouth breathing during sleep. All-day symptoms require further evaluation. Older children can obtain relief by using sucking candies or throat lozenges.

Although children remain contagious during the entire course of a runny nose, most can *return to school* when they have been without fever for 24 hours (temperature less than 101°F [38.4°C]); if they have only occasional coughing; and if they appear well. During early school years, children may average one or two colds a month, and parents find that it is not practical for the children to remain at home until they are completely well.

Wheezing (Asthma, Asthmatic Bronchitis, Hyperactive Airway Disease, "Wheezy" Bronchitis, Bronchiolitis)

Screening Questions

Background
- Name, age, sex?
- Chronic illness?
- Current medications and treatments?

Duration
- How long has wheezing been present?

Past History
- Has the child had wheezing or asthma in the past?
- If yes, does the older child use a peak flow meter?

Quality of Wheezing
- Is wheezing present only when the child breathes out or when the child breathes in and out?

Difficulty Breathing
- Does the child have to strain or work hard to get air in and out?
- Is the child's chest heaving while breathing?
- Does the child have poor (dusky or bluish) skin color?
- If the child uses a peak flow meter, is the child cooperative while using the meter? How do current peak flow (peak expiratory flow rate, PEFR) readings compare to the child's personal-best baseline? What has been the response to treatment?

Fever
- If fever is present, how high is it and when did it begin?

Other Symptoms
- Are cold or other symptoms present?
- Does the child have a barking cough or hoarse voice?

Emergencies
and Traumas

Minor
Infections

Infectious
Diseases

Parenting
Concerns

Infant
Care

Jeffrey L. Brown: *Pediatric Telephone Medicine: Principles, Triage, and Advice,*
Second Edition. Copyright © 1994 J. B. Lippincott Company

General
Principles

Common
Symptoms

Emergencies
and Traumas

Minor
Infections

Infectious
Diseases

Parenting
Concerns

Infant
Care

General Appearance

■ Does the child look especially sick?

Examine Immediately If

- The child looks toxic.
- The child is less than 3 months old and has been wheezing for more than 1 hour.
- The child has wheezing or has to strain or work hard to get air in and out after medication has been given.
- The child has poor skin color.
- A symptomatic child's peak flow remains less than 50% of the personal-best baseline (in the red zone) after adequate treatment.

Examine in the Near Future If

- Symptoms last longer than 8 hours.
- Temperature is greater than 101°F (38.4°C) for longer than 24 hours.
- Peak flow remains between 80% and 50% of the personal-best baseline (in the yellow zone) after adequate treatment.

See Related Sections

The toxic child (p. 61), cough (p. 65), upper respiratory infection (p. 81), croup (p. 69), fever (p. 53).

Treatment

- Sitting or semisitting position.
- Humidified air if symptoms are associated with mouth breathing.
- Oral or inhaled bronchodilators when these are available.
- Decongestants if wheezing is associated with an upper respiratory tract infection.
- Antihistamines if severe upper respiratory allergic symptoms are present.
- Clear liquids offered frequently, especially when the child has been eating or drinking poorly.
- Air-conditioned room for allergic children during summer months.

Parent Call-back Is Needed for

- Persistent, changing, worsening, anxiety-provoking, or specific symptoms as outlined above.

Discussion

Parents of children with known *hyperactive airway disease* may call for reassurance during acute attacks even when they have mastered successful treatment strategies. When *bronchodilators* or other medicines have already been given to treat an acute attack but symptoms are still present, carefully review dosage and frequency of administration to confirm that both are appropriate for the child's age and size. Treatment failures may be related to errors of underdosing. *Antihistamines* may be useful for children with allergy-induced illness. Some medicine package inserts still describe antihistamines as contraindicated for asthmatics because they may thicken tracheal and bronchial secretions; this effect appears to be minimal if it occurs at all. Similarly, *decongestants* may also be helpful when sneezing and rhinitis have precipitated the attack.

Hydration can sometimes decrease mucous viscosity in a dehydrated patient, but overhydration is not beneficial and may make the patient worse. Since medicines for wheezing and wheezing itself can both induce nausea and vomiting, fluid intake should also be reviewed.

Wheezing tends to begin or worsen at *nighttime*. Bedroom *allergens* can sometimes precipitate symptoms, but when the symptoms don't occur during daytime naps in the same room, bronchospasm is more likely to reflect changes in temperature, humidity, or body cycle. *Air conditioners* should be set to recirculate during warm weather months to help control these changes and to decrease pollen entry through open windows. Attic fans should be avoided since they draw irritants and pollen directly into the house. *Humidifiers* are easily contaminated with mold and may be harmful for allergic children. An open pot of water in a dry heated room is a useful substitute.

Any *irritant* may worsen symptoms, but cigarette smoking is the most common offender and should be strictly avoided. Other substances that may cause lung irritation include menthol-containing medicines that are rubbed on the patients' chest or added to hot steam vaporizers.

Wheezing associated with fever and cough suggests the presence of active *infection.* Most infection-induced wheezing episodes are viral in origin, but antibiotic therapy may sometimes be indicated. Children younger than 9 months old who have been wheezing more than a few hours should be suspected of having viral *bronchiolitis. Allergic triggers* should be looked for when there is a strong positive family history of al-

General
Principles

Common
Symptoms

Emergencies
and Traumas

Minor
Infections

Infectious
Diseases

Parenting
Concerns

Infant
Care

lergy or other allergic symptoms. *Hospitalization* may become necessary for worsening symptoms when home treatment has been ineffective. Parental anxiety, fatigue, and loss of objectivity may also make inpatient care necessary.

> **CLINICAL TIP.** The wheezing heard when a child has *croup* (laryngeotracheobronchitis) is usually associated with a barking cough and hoarse voice and is present on both *inspiration and expiration;* wheezing from bronchospasm is usually heard only on expiration.

When older children have chronic or frequently recurring symptoms, home use of inexpensive *peak flow meters* can be a valuable aid for the successful management of hyperactive airway disease. Objective assessment of pulmonary function encourages early intervention and allows for optimal adjustment of medication on an as-needed basis. But it is important to evaluate the *reliability* of peak flow (peak expiratory flow rate, PEFR) readings before they are used to make decisions that will affect triage and treatment. Inaccurate "personal-best" baseline measurements might minimize the later effects of bronchospasm. Unreliable readings taken when the child is ill will most commonly overestimate the severity of an acute illness: An otherwise cooperative child might lack the motivation or be unable to use her meter properly while experiencing symptoms such as headache, nausea, or vomiting. And peak flow measured in the supine or sitting position might be useful for establishing a trend, but should not be compared to a baseline obtained when the child is standing. Frequent obvious discrepancies between clinical observations and peak flow readings suggest a need to reevaluate the patient's attitude, aptitude, and technique.

Parents calling to report changes in peak flow should have already followed individualized instructions issued earlier based on the child's previous pattern of illness. For example, the mother might have been told that inhaled bronchodilators are not needed during a respiratory illness when readings are higher than 80% of the child's personal-best baseline level (sometimes designated as being in the green zone); but to give treatments every 4 to 6 hours if they drop to between 80% and 50% of the personal-best level (the yellow zone); and to give up to three treatments 1 hour apart and then call if they remain lower than 50% of personal-best level (the red zone).

Parents are commonly confused by the different medicines used to treat asthma and by the different triggers that may precipitate symptoms.

Whenever there have been multiple episodes of wheezing, *education of the parent* and the child (depending on age) should be considered mandatory. These discussions should be scheduled as a formal conference, but sometimes an abbreviated version over the telephone is needed to relieve anxiety and improve parental objectivity during the acute attack. Telephoned conversations during acute attacks should be heavily weighted toward recognizing signs and symptoms of worsening illness and the proper administration of medicines, but brief mention of other pertinent topics may be appropriate depending on circumstance. Topics for discussion might include:

1. *Etiology.* Wheezing occurs when irritable or twitchy airways become constricted from infection, exercise, allergy, anxiety or irritants in any combination. The wheezing or whistling sound is caused by air pushed through narrowed bronchial tubes when the child breathes out. Irritation inside the narrow airway can also cause difficulty breathing or coughing.

2. *Signs of worsening illness.* Parents should be more concerned about the child's general appearance and the amount of effort needed to breathe than about wheezing noises made while breathing. Sometimes decreased wheezing means that the child is getting worse rather than better: Less airflow may decrease the wheezing noise. Warning signs of worsening illness include straining or "pulling" to breathe, rapid short breaths, grunting while breathing, poor color, and an ill general appearance.

CLINICAL TIP. Experienced parents can learn to recognize early signs of bronchospasm without peak flow meters or other similar devices by simply watching for a reversed inspiratory/expiratory breathing pattern: A child normally takes longer to breathe air in than to breathe air out; bronchospasm causes the reverse. Early intervention, before wheezing occurs, may be used at that point to avoid a more serious wheezing attack.

3. *Treatment.* Oral bronchodilating agents may be helpful to reopen the airways of small wheezing children, or they may be used for prolonged action in older children. Inhaled bronchodilators using a nebulizer or metered dose inhaler (MDI) with a spacing chamber are preferred because of rapid onset of action and fewer side effects. These can include tremulousness, rapid heart beat, nausea, and vomiting. When bronchodilators are needed frequently, inhaled and oral steroids and other medicines may also be re-

General Principles

Common Symptoms

Emergencies and Traumas

Minor Infections

Infectious Diseases

Parenting Concerns

Infant Care

General
Principles

Common
Symptoms

Emergencies
and Traumas

Minor
Infections

Infectious
Diseases

Parenting
Concerns

Infant
Care

quired to reduce airway inflammation that can lead to spasm. The most common immediate treatment for an acute wheezing attack is to increase the dose or frequency of bronchodilating medicine. Parents should be able to distinguish between medicines used to prevent and to treat attacks and between those used to decrease airway spasm and to decrease airway inflammation. They should also know that the same medication may be labeled with two or three different brand names.

CLINICAL TIP. When spacers are not available for MDIs, a paper cup with a hole made at the base creates a useful mask for small children through which medicated mist can be sprayed; a plastic soda bottle with a hole made at the base can be used as a temporary spacing chamber for older children.

4. *Prevention.* Known precipitating factors should be avoided whenever practical. Mold and dust control should be practiced; pets should be suspect; cigarette smoke should be prohibited; and a search should be made for other agents that may worsen symptoms. These include perfumes contained in soap, shampoo, and laundry detergent. Medicine may also be administered prophylactically on a daily basis for frequent attacks or on an as-needed basis for activities or situations known to cause wheezing, such as exercise.

5. *Review.* At the conclusion of the telephoned discussion, the parent should understand which medicines should be used and how often they should be given; under what circumstances to call for further advice; and that further teaching sessions are needed to clarify long-range objectives.

General
Principles

Common
Symptoms

Emergencies
and Traumas

Minor
Infections

Infectious
Diseases

Parenting
Concerns

Infant
Care

Abdominal Pain in Older Children

Screening Questions

Background
- Name, age, sex?
- Chronic illness?
- Current medications and treatments?

Duration
- How long have symptoms been present?

Fever
- If fever is present, how high is it and when did it begin?

Trauma
- Was there injury to the abdomen before the onset of symptoms?

Duration
- How long has pain been present?

Location
- Is the pain generalized, localized mostly to the area around the belly button, or is it worst at another location?

Bowel Movements
- Does the child have constipation, diarrhea, or bloody bowel movements?

Vomiting
- If there has been vomiting, when did it begin and how often has the child thrown up?

Exposure
- Has the child had recent exposure to others with similar symptoms?

General
Principles

Common
Symptoms

Emergencies
and Traumas

Minor
Infections

Infectious
Diseases

Parenting
Concerns

Infant
Care

Other Symptoms

■ Does the child have other symptoms including rash or painful or frequent urination?

General Appearance

■ Does the child look especially sick?

Examine Immediately If

- The child appears toxic.
- Pain is localized to the lower abdomen (regardless of side) and remains localized for more than 2 hours.
- Grossly bloody stools are present.
- Green or bile-stained vomitus is noted on multiple occasions.

Examine in the Near Future If

- Pain lasts longer than 24 hours.
- Temperature is greater than 101°F (38.4°C) for more than 24 hours.
- Urinary symptoms are present.

See Related Sections

The toxic child (p. 61), diarrhea (p. 107), constipation (p. 97), vomiting (p. 111), fever (p. 53), urinary tract infection (p. 121).

Treatment

- Clear liquid diet for 2 hours followed by a bland diet until symptoms disappear. (See p. 274.)
- Heating pad applied to the abdomen for older children if it provides relief.
- Consider use of antispasmodic medicines.
- Consider symptomatic treatment of diarrhea or constipation.

Parent Call-back Is Needed for

- Persistent, changing, worsening, anxiety-provoking, or specific symptoms as outlined above.

Discussion

- *Acute appendicitis* is the most common cause of surgically important abdominal pain in older children. Children *5 years old and older* with appendicitis typically have a history that includes low-grade temperature, loss of appetite, and worsening periumbilical pain that gradually becomes more intense and localized to the lower abdomen, especially on the right side. There may be some change in stooling pattern, and vomiting is frequently present. The younger the child, the less frequent is the condition, and the more likely the presentation will be atypical. In the early stages, *younger children* may have symptoms and physical findings that mimic a simple gastroenteritis. Asking questions that pertain to the child's general appearance and maintaining a reasonable index of suspicion is the best one can do to recognize this frequently missed diagnosis.

- *Trauma* to the abdomen may result in a ruptured viscus. Sledding accidents are among the most common to cause a ruptured liver or spleen. Evaluation is required when the child complains of pain together with a pale or shocky appearance.
- *Nonsurgical abdominal pain* is the most likely diagnosis when other family members have similar symptoms, when the pain is localized to the umbilicus (the child points to the belly button when asked where the stomach hurts most), or when nonbilious vomiting and/or nonbloody diarrheal stools are present. Viral *gastroenteritis* and gas pains are usually self-limited and can be treated expectantly or symptomatically.

> **CLINICAL TIP.** It is best to evaluate the child's general appearance when there have been no active cramps or vomiting for 15 or 20 minutes. It is also wise to ask parents to have the child get out of bed to walk around. Frequently, the child's gait will appear normal and he will seem better. Children who are vomiting or nauseated look pale, sweaty, and "toxic" but improve shortly after the vomiting or nausea disappears. When the child looks well, there is less chance that serious illness is present.

- *Intussusception* is an exception to the above rule. When one portion of the bowel telescopes over the other, resulting obstruction causes spasms of severe pain at 15- or 20-minute intervals. The child may look extremely ill during spasms but show marked improvement during rest periods. This diagnosis should be suspected when a child between the ages of a few months and 3 years has short bouts of intermittent pain together with vomiting and bloody, jelly-like ("currant jelly") stools.

- *Urinary symptoms* can sometimes be associated with abdominal pain, especially when an obstructive uropathy is present.
- *Rashes* associated with colicky abdominal pain are relatively uncommon. These include the hemorrhagic rash on the lower extremities and buttocks in patients with Henoch-Schönlein syndrome and rashes on light-exposed areas of the body as seen in patients with porphyria.
- *Chronic and recurrent abdominal pain* has a long list of potential causes, and thorough evaluation is needed even when the history suggests that it is *psychogenic* in origin.

CLINICAL TIP. Children with frequent symptoms of both psychogenic and organic etiology are more likely to complain when they are looking for attention or when they are stressed even though symptoms may be present all day.

- *Lactose* and other forms of *carbohydrate intolerance* are commonly missed as causes of recurrent pain: The symptoms may be dose-related, but in some children very small amounts of these sugars can cause symptoms. Lactose intolerance or cow milk allergy should be suspected if there is a strong family history for this condition or if there was cow milk intolerance or colic in early infancy. (See p. 104.) Use the milk-free diet given in the appendix as a therapeutic trial. *Apple juice* drinkers frequently complain of cramps, gas, and loose stools, and children who drink large amounts of soda may be *fructose* intolerant; symptoms disappear when they change to diet soda. Those chewing "sugarless" gum or eating "sugarless" candies may also be malabsorbing nondigestible sugars. Diet manipulation is inexpensive and noninvasive and may be discussed over the phone before the child is brought to the office for a complete examination.

General
Principles

Common
Symptoms

Emergencies
and Traumas

Minor
Infections

Infectious
Diseases

Parenting
Concerns

Infant
Care

CLINICAL TIP. The most common error when prescribing these diets is to assume that small quantities of milk products contained in baked goods and other foods will not cause symptoms.

Learn sample clear-liquid and bland diets so that these can be presented to the parent by rote when the child has simple gastroenteritis. (See p. 274.)

Constipation

Screening Questions

Background
- Name, age, sex?
- Chronic illness?
- Current medications including vitamins and iron?

Frequency
- How often does your child have a bowel movement?

Consistency
- Are stools hard or soft?

Duration
- When did the constipation first begin?

Blood
- Is blood mixed with or streaked on stools?

Other Findings
- Is there tender redness around the child's rectal opening?

Past History
- Does your child have a past history of constipation?

Examine Immediately

- Rarely necessary.

Examine in the Near Future If

- Blood-streaked stools occur on more than one occasion.
- There is a history of chronic or recurrent symptoms.
- The perianal area is red or tender to touch.

Jeffrey L. Brown: *Pediatric Telephone Medicine: Principles, Triage, and Advice*,
Second Edition. Copyright © 1994 J. B. Lippincott Company

General
Principles

Common
Symptoms

Emergencies
and Traumas

Minor
Infections

Infectious
Diseases

Parenting
Concerns

Infant
Care

Treatment

Infants

- Initial rectal stimulation with a thermometer or infant-sized glycerin suppository.
- Add sugar or malt-sugar extract to formula or water, ½ teaspoonful to 4 ounces for at least 3 days.
- Prune juice, 1 to 3 ounces, diluted with equal parts of water if there is no change.
- For chronic symptoms, try soy or protein hydrolysate formula for a least 1 week.

Older Children

- For initial treatment, use a prepackaged enema.
- Later, use a mild laxative, such as milk of magnesia, senna, or mineral oil in decreasing doses to promote daily stooling and to keep the stool soft for at least 2- to 3-week periods.
- For chronic constipation, use laxatives and/or stool softeners together with increased fiber to keep stools soft for at least 6 weeks. Resume treatment for recurrence.

Parent Call-back Is Needed for

- Persistent, changing, worsening, anxiety-provoking, or specific symptoms as outlined above.

Discussion

Constipation of short duration is of little medical significance except for transient distress while passing a hard stool. A glycerine suppository or a prepackaged enema together with much reassurance will usually provide prompt symptomatic relief.

CLINICAL TIP. The most frequently made mistake while treating *chronic constipation* is to use laxatives for too short a period of time. "Laxative dependency" is rarely a problem for small children.

A common pattern leading to constipation in young children is a delay in stooling because of resistance to toilet training, lack of a conve-

nient toilet or potty, dietary change, poor fluid intake, laziness, or oppositional behavior. Resultant hard stools cause painful defecation and possible rectal fissure (suggested by blood streaking on the stool). Fear of
pain creates reluctance to defecate at the next urge, and resulting hard
stool again causes painful defecation, which repeats the cycle.

Once symptoms have continued for weeks or months, they can be relieved only by changing the child's habit pattern over a prolonged period
of time. Initial treatment should consist of eliminating hard stool with an
enema or laxative and then keeping stools permanently soft by using the
smallest dose of laxative necessary to maintain stool consistency at
slightly harder than runny. The dose should also be high enough to make
it impossible for the child to withhold stool voluntarily. Occasionally
prune juice or stool softeners may be effective for chronic constipation,
but laxatives are usually necessary. Laxative dose should be tapered slowly at 2-week intervals but returned to the previous higher levels if hard
stools recur.

Allowing time for defecation, especially after large meals, assuring
adequate fluid intake, and temporarily eliminating toilet training when
the child has shown strong resistance may also be useful. A careful dietary history should be taken. Drinking large quantities of milk, eating
foods too low in fiber, or taking vitamin supplements high in iron may be
contributing factors. Iron-containing infant formulas are only occasionally responsible for symptoms, but for an occasional infant, a trial of iron-
free formula can be dramatically successful. Older children may also require behavior modification techniques with verbal or other rewards for
good stooling practices; little attention together with a firm negative directive should be used for failure.

Perianal redness or tenderness suggests the possibility of *streptococcal infection* that may require antibiotic treatment. Chronic symptoms unresponsive to simple measures require complete evaluation, especially
when they began during early infancy.

Common
Symptoms

Emergencies
and Traumas

Minor
Infections

Infectious
Diseases

Parenting
Concerns

Infant
Care

Prolonged or Recurrent Infant Crying (Infant Colic, Abdominal Pain in Infants)

Screening Questions

Background
- Name, age, sex?
- Chronic illness?
- Current medications and treatments?
- Recent immunizations?

Duration
- How long have symptoms been present?

Frequency
- How often do severe bouts of crying occur?

Fever
- If fever is present, how high is it and when did it begin?

Feeding
- Has the baby been feeding and sucking normally?
- Has the baby been taking breast milk, formula, or solids?

Vomiting
- If the baby has been throwing up, how frequent is the vomiting and how long has it been going on?
- Is the vomit green?

Bowel Movements
- How frequent is the baby's stooling and what is its consistency?
- When was the baby's last bowel movement?
- If blood is present on stooling, is it mixed throughout the stool or is it just streaked on the surface?

Other Signs and Symptoms
- When the baby is completely undressed, is there swelling in the groin or other parts of the body, tearing or redness in one eye, unusual rash, or any other finding of concern?

Jeffrey L. Brown: *Pediatric Telephone Medicine: Principles, Triage, and Advice,*
Second Edition. Copyright © 1994 J. B. Lippincott Company

General
Principles

Common
Symptoms

Emergencies
and Traumas

Minor
Infections

Infectious
Diseases

Parenting
Concerns

Infant
Care

General Appearance
■ Does the baby look especially sick?

Examine Immediately If

- The baby looks toxic.
- Bile-stained vomit is present on multiple occasions.
- Grossly bloody diarrhea is present (not occasional blood streaking).
- The baby has refused the last three feedings.
- Fever has been present for more than 4 hours.

Examine in the near Future If

- Cramps continue for more than 3 to 4 hours per day.

See Related Sections

The toxic child (p. 61), vomiting (p. 111), diarrhea (p. 107), fever (p. 53).

Treatment

- Initial diet change to clear liquids.
- Symptomatic treatment of constipation if present.
- Much reassurance if the suspected diagnosis is infant colic.

Parent Call-back Is Needed for

- Persistent, changing, worsening, anxiety-provoking, or specific symptoms as outlined above.

Discussion

Infants described as appearing pale, sweaty, apprehensive, or extremely ill for more than 30 minutes should be examined at the earliest possible time. Those crying because of teething, colic, gas pains, or recent immunizations, especially diphtheria, pertussis, tetanus (DPT) shots, usually look reasonably well during the crying episodes.

CLINICAL TIP. All children with uncontrolled crying should be completely undressed at home to look for causes other than "colic". Some of these are listed below.
- *Corneal abrasion* is suggested when there is a single eye that is red or tearing.
- *Incarcerated hernia* is suggested when there is tender inguinal or scrotal swelling.
- *Circulatory obstruction* can occur when a thread or hair inadvertently becomes wrapped around a toe, a finger, or the penis.
- *Missed trauma* can sometimes be detected when swelling is noted over a single collarbone or other body part.
- *Severe diaper rash* with open and oozing sores can sometimes cause prolonged crying.

- *Constipation* should be suspected when infants have a history of frequent, hard stools associated with straining. Crying usually occurs only at the time of stooling. Blood streaking on the stool may indicate the presence of a fissure. A bright red perianal area might be caused by streptococcal cellulitis, which will respond to oral antibiotics.
- *Gastroesophageal reflux* is present to some degree in most healthy infants. Esophageal irritation and colicky symptoms sometimes can result. Treatment using head-up prone positioning after eating, cereal-thickened feedings, and oral antacids may prove of value.
- *Infection,* especially of the ear and urinary tract, can cause prolonged crying, and some babies with central nervous system involvement may not be pacified by usual handling and feeding techniques. Fever and ill appearance may be present. An occasional association of crying while voiding or with ear-pulling may be obvious.
- *Intestinal obstruction* should be suspected when infants have more than one episode of green-stained vomit. Grossly bloody diarrhea should also prompt early examination. Some infants will have simple *gastroenteritis,* but an abdominal condition that requires surgery can be ruled out only by thorough examination. Occasional blood streaking mixed with mucous can be caused by a variety of bowel irritants and by cow milk allergy.

General Principles

Common Symptoms

Emergencies and Traumas

Minor Infections

Infectious Diseases

Parenting Concerns

Infant Care

General
Principles

Common
Symptoms

Emergencies
and Traumas

Minor
Infections

Infectious
Diseases

Parenting
Concerns

Infant
Care

Evaluation should not be considered emergent unless the child is described as appearing ill.

- *Overfeeding* can lead to abdominal cramping, loose stools, and spitting up.

> **CLINICAL TIP.** An approximation of the number of ounces of combined food and milk tolerated at one feeding can be made by halving the baby's weight in pounds and adding ±1. Thus, a 14-pound infant would average 7 ounces per feeding and can tolerate 6 to 8 ounces as a combination of food and milk.

- *Air swallowing* by rapid-feeders can result in abdominal distention and distress. Frequent allowances for burping and propping the baby after nursing may be of some help. However, crying babies tend to burp when picked up because of swallowed air; their crying may then be attributed to gas pains rather than the reverse.
- *Cow milk intolerance* or milk allergy should be presumed when symptoms are relieved after a 5-day trial of soy or protein hydrolysate formula or after a nursing mother is placed on a cow milk-product-free diet. If there is no change in symptoms, the infant should be returned to a standard milk formula. This diagnosis should especially be suspected in black and Jewish infants and in those with a strong family history of milk intolerance or spastic colon. Cow milk allergy can be seen in breast-fed babies also since offending cow milk proteins cross into breast milk.
- *Infant colic* is the term used to describe babies who have prolonged crying episodes and appear to be in greater distress than is expected of most other babies. As with hyperactivity in older children, there is a subjective element to this diagnosis, but some of these infants are clearly different from most other babies. During crying episodes they may appear flushed, draw up their knees, and strain. Typically, severe crying bouts last more than 4 hours and occur more frequently than three times per week. These infants may get only transient relief while feeding (although they may appear to be hungry), cuddling, or sucking. Colic usually begins during the first week of life and improves at about 3 months of age. Crying bouts that are limited to the early evening hours are referred to as *night colic*. In most cases, a definite cause will not be found. Advising parents at pre- and postnatal visits that normal and healthy babies can cry 3 to 6 hours a day during the first few

weeks can be helpful toward relieving anxiety and changing expectations.

- *Treatment strategies* include changing formulas, using different nipples and bottles, eliminating foods from breast-feeding mothers' diets (especially cow milk products and xanthines such as caffeine and chocolate), using simethacone drops or herbal teas, using mechanical rocking devices (including long car rides), experimenting with demand vs. strict feeding schedules, and increasing or decreasing infant "cuddle time." All of these approaches have professional and nonprofessional proponents, opponents, and those who are neutral. At their request, allow parents of colicky babies to try any strategy that is safe; all seem to work for some individual babies. Most parents can be helped by reassurance and education once food allergy is ruled out.

General
Principles

Common
Symptoms

Emergencies
and Traumas

Minor
Infections

Infectious
Diseases

Parenting
Concerns

Infant
Care

Diarrhea

Screening Questions

Background
- Name, age, sex?
- Chronic illness?
- Current medications and treatments?

Duration
- When did the diarrhea begin?

Frequency
- How often does stooling occur?

Description
- Are bowel movements large or small?
- Do stools contain blood?
- If yes, is it mixed or just streaked throughout the stool?

Fever
- If fever is present, when did it begin and how high is it?

Gastrointestinal Symptoms
- Does the child have vomiting or stomach cramps?

Other Symptoms
- Are there other symptoms such as earache, runny nose, or rash?

Hydration
- Has the child been eating or drinking?
- If this is a younger child, does she cry with tears?
- Does the child make urine at regular intervals?

Contacts
- Has there been recent exposure to others with stomach cramps, vomiting, diarrhea, or fever?

General Appearance
- Does the child look especially sick?

Jeffrey L. Brown: *Pediatric Telephone Medicine: Principles, Triage, and Advice*, Second Edition. Copyright © 1994 J. B. Lippincott Company

107

General
Principles

Common
Symptoms

Emergencies
and Traumas

Minor
Infections

Infectious
Diseases

Parenting
Concerns

Infant
Care

Examine Immediately If

- The child appears toxic.
- An infant is believed to have significant dehydration especially when vomiting is present and the child is lethargic.
- Severe abdominal pain is present.

Examine in the Near Future If

- Diarrhea has lasted longer than 3 days.
- Associated vomiting has lasted longer than 24 hours.
- Temperature greater than 101°F (38.4°C) has lasted longer than 24 hours.
- Stools are grossly bloody.
- Symptoms are worse following treatment.

See Related Sections

The toxic child (p. 61), vomiting (p. 111), abdominal cramps in older children (p. 91), crying in infants (p. 101), fever (p. 53).

Treatment

Infants Less Than 1 Year Old
- Small, frequent feedings with a commercial electrolyte solution for 4 to 8 hours, then
- One-half strength formula (soy, lactose-free, or protein hydrolysate may be preferred) for 12 to 24 hours, then
- Full-strength formula, then
- Add strained banana, rice, and apple sauce if the infant previously has been taking solids and if full-strength formula is tolerated.
- When primary or secondary lactose intolerance is suspected, avoid giving milk or milk products until bowel movements have been normal for 3 to 4 days.
- If breast-fed, the infant should be given small, frequent feedings of electrolyte solution for 4 to 8 hours while the mother expresses breast milk manually. If there is dehydration, breast feedings may require supplementation with small amounts of water or electrolyte solution between feedings.

Children Over 1 Year Old
- Diet should avoid milk and milk products or lactose-reduced products should be used if lactose intolerance is suspected.
- Clear liquids with bland foods should be given.

- Antispasmodics may be useful for cramping.
- Consider use of absorbents such as activated attapulgite or medicines such as bismuth subsalicylate.

Parent Call-back Is Needed for

- Persistent, changing, worsening, anxiety-provoking, or specific symptoms as outlined above.

Discussion

Clarification of history is necessary before establishing the need for a complex treatment regimen: Parents may report "terrible diarrhea" when the child has passed a single loose stool that has soiled the child's clothing. Both infants and older children who have passed only a few diarrheal stools require little more than expectant treatment.

- *Infant diarrhea* can be confused with *normal infant stools,* which can be runny, pasty or mucous, especially when the baby is breast-fed. Also many babies stool with each feeding and occasionally in between. Unless true diarrheal stools have been noted consecutively on three or four occasions, no treatment is necessary. While on clear liquids, stools may remain watery since no solids are being ingested. If the infant is changed to a soy formula, stools may assume a pasty consistency and gray-green color.
- *Dehydration* can be difficult to evaluate over the telephone. Small infants with normal hydration may cry without tears, urine is frequently mixed with runny stools, and mouth-breathing may make mucous membranes appear dry. For these reasons, a child's activity level and general appearance must substitute for degree of hydration when triage decisions are made.
- *Oral rehydrating electrolyte solutions* have been extremely effective at decreasing the incidence of seriously dehydrated babies and for treating dehydration once it occurs. One must be certain that oral intake exceeds diarrheal outflow. Small, frequent feedings make vomiting less likely, and occasionally spoon feedings of electrolyte solutions may be necessary. Solutions should be given to the baby at a rate of about 5 ml (1 teaspoon) per minute up to 10 ounces per hour, or more slowly if the baby is throwing up.

CLINICAL TIP. Commercial electrolyte solutions are safest because preparation is virtually error-free. However, home remedies may be required when these are not available. An effective substitute can be prepared by mixing 1 cup of dry precooked baby rice

General Principles

Common Symptoms

Emergencies and Traumas

Minor Infections

Infectious Diseases

Parenting Concerns

Infant Care

General Principles

Common Symptoms

Emergencies and Traumas

Minor Infections

Infectious Diseases

Parenting Concerns

Infant Care

cereal with 1 quart of cool boiled or bottled water and a carefully measured $\frac{1}{2}$ teaspoon of salt.

- *Boiled skim milk* should *never* be used to treat infant diarrhea. Evaporation of water during boiling increases lactose concentration, which can cause malabsorption, and increased sodium content can cause dangerous hypernatremia.
- Protect the infant's bottom with zinc oxide or a similar ointment since *diaper rash* is likely to follow any prolonged bout of diarrhea.
- *Older children with diarrhea* do not require the meticulous treatment regimen employed for infants. However, even they can develop dehydration, and evaluation is certainly required when they appear ill.
- *Dietary management* consists of clear liquids to replace and prevent further fluid losses, early introduction of bland foods, which can include boiled chicken, potatoes, eggs, and pasta, as well as banana, apple sauce, toast, and cereal.
- *Medications* are not usually needed to treat the diarrhea of younger children. Activated attapulgite is safe and may thicken stools and decrease frequency, but as an absorbent it can also absorb out other medicines given at the same time. Bismuth subsalicylate appears to be effective at proper doses. But there is some concern about the safety of salicylates given during viral illness, and unless prewarned, parents can become apprehensive when this medicine turns stools and the tongue black. Trimethoprim-sulfamethoxizole is thought by many to be useful for treating "traveller's diarrhea," and if used should be continued for some days after symptoms have resolved. Opiate derivatives may decrease cramping as well as diarrhea but are not generally recommended because dose levels needed for efficacy approach toxicity. Antibiotics may be required to treat diarrhea caused by pathogenic bacteria or parasites. Further evaluation is needed for chronic or recurrent symptoms and for diarrhea associated with grossly bloody stools, high fever, severe abdominal cramps, and weight loss.

CLINICAL TIP. When offering foods and liquids to children with severe diarrhea, make special effort to reduce the disaccharide sugar content when practical: lactose-reduced milk is preferred to regular milk, canned fruits should have the sweet syrups removed before serving, and juices should be diluted with water.

General
Principles

Common
Symptoms

Emergencies
and Traumas

Minor
Infections

Infectious
Diseases

Parenting
Concerns

Infant
Care

Vomiting (Emesis)

Screening Questions

Background
- Name, age, sex?
- Chronic illness?
- Current medications and treatments?

Duration
- When did the vomiting begin?

Frequency
- How often does the child throw up?
- Is vomiting present with all or only some feedings or meals?

Fever
- If fever is present, how high is it and when did it begin?

Gastrointestinal Symptoms
- Is abdominal pain present at a time different from the time of vomiting?
- Does the child have diarrhea or constipation?

Trauma
- Did the vomiting follow trauma to the head or abdomen?

Other Symptoms
- Are other symptoms or findings such as sore throat, earache, severe headache, or rash present?
- Are neurological symptoms such as incoordination or confusion present?

Hydration
- If this is a small child, does he cry with tears and does he pass urine at regular intervals?

Jeffrey L. Brown: *Pediatric Telephone Medicine: Principles, Triage, and Advice,* Second Edition. Copyright © 1994 J. B. Lippincott Company

General
Principles

Common
Symptoms

Emergencies
and Traumas

Minor
Infections

Infectious
Diseases

Parenting
Concerns

Infant
Care

Contacts

■ Was there recent exposure to others with stomach pain, vomiting, diarrhea, or fever?

General Appearance

■ Does the child look especially sick?

Examine Immediately If

- The child has neurological signs or symptoms, especially following trauma or if associated with high fever.
- The child appears toxic.

Examine in the Near Future If

- Vomiting lasts longer than 12 hours.
- The child does not cry with tears or urinate at regular intervals, especially when copious diarrhea is present.

See Related Sections

The toxic child (p. 61), abdominal pain in older children (p. 91), infant crying (p. 101), diarrhea (p. 107), fever (p. 53), trauma to the head (p. 141), trauma to the abdomen (p. 91).

Treatment

- Clear liquids offered in small frequent amounts until there has been no vomiting for 4 hours, followed by a soft, bland diet. (See p. 274.)
- Acetaminophen rectal suppositories for a symptomatic febrile child who is unable to retain oral medication.

Parent Call-back Is Needed for

- Persistent, changing, worsening, anxiety-provoking, or specific symptoms as outlined above.

Discussion

Vomiting is a *nonspecific* symptom that can be associated with many illnesses and conditions ranging from migraine headache to ingestion of foreign substances. Most episodes are caused by simple *viral gastroenteritis.* Suspect this diagnosis when a family member has had recent intestinal symptoms, the child has crampy abdominal pain that occurs just prior to vomiting, or when vomiting is associated with loose or diarrheal stools.

Deviation from this history should make the clinician suspicious of other causes: High fever may be associated with *infection* such as streptococcal pharyngitis or otitis; extreme lethargy may suggest other illnesses, including meningitis; and persistent bile-staining of vomitus or prolonged abdominal pain between bouts of vomiting is consistent with an abdominal condition requiring surgery. A history of past frequent episodes of vomiting warrants a complete history and physical examination, although not necessarily on an emergency basis.

Dehydration does not usually occur in an otherwise healthy child unless there is also fluid loss from copious diarrhea or symptoms have been present for more than 48 hours. *Abdominal pain* should be considered significant when it occurs at times other than when the child is vomiting.

Vomiting associated with *central nervous system* (CNS) *symptoms* (change in level of consciousness, incoordination, or headache) requires early examination. When vomiting and CNS symptoms follow a recent antecedent viral illness such as influenza or chickenpox, consider the possibility of *Reye's syndrome,* especially if the child has received aspirin.

Instruct parents to offer *clear liquids* in small and frequent amounts: one-half fruit-juice-sized glass every 20 minutes. Immediately after vomiting, the child may feel thirsty, drink a large quantity of fluid, and vomit again. Commercial electrolyte solutions are useful for younger children and infants. If carbonated beverages are chosen, they should be stirred to remove as much gas as possible. Diet sodas and plain water should be avoided because they lack calories. Fruit juice mixed to one-half strength with water, weak tea with sugar, clear broth, or gelatin desert may also be used in clear liquid diets.

General Principles

Common Symptoms

Emergencies and Traumas

Minor Infections

Infectious Diseases

Parenting Concerns

Infant Care

113

Headache

Screening Questions

Background
- Name, age, sex?
- Chronic illness?
- Current medications and treatments?

Duration
- How long have symptoms been present?

Severity
- Is the pain severe enough to interfere with usual activities?

Fever
- If fever is present, how high is it and when did it begin?

Trauma
- Did the child hit or hurt her head before the onset of symptoms?

Other General Symptoms
- Does the child have other symptoms such as upper respiratory infection, allergic symptoms (itchy eyes or nose), nausea, or vomiting?

Central Nervous System (CNS) Symptoms
- Does the child have incoordination, difficulty with speech, confusion, or excessive sleepiness?

Symptom Pattern
- Have there been other episodes of headache recently?
- Is the pain usually at the same location of the head?
- How long do headaches usually last?
- Do they awaken the child from sleep, occur early in the morning, or seem to occur at the same time every day?
- Do headaches seem to occur while performing any particular activity?
- What seems to make the headache better?

General
Principles

Common
Symptoms

Emergencies
and Traumas

Minor
Infections

Infectious
Diseases

Parenting
Concerns

Infant
Care

Family History

■ Is there a family history of recurrent headache or migraine?

General Appearance

■ Does the child look especially sick?

Examine Immediately If

- The child appears toxic.
- There is extreme parental anxiety.
- The headache is severe and has occurred after head trauma.
- The headache is associated with other CNS symptoms.

Examine in the Near Future If

- There are recurrent symptoms that interfere with the child's activity.
- There are associated symptoms that suggest acute or chronic illness.

See Related Sections

The toxic child (p. 61), head trauma (p. 141), upper respiratory infection (p. 81), and fever (p. 53).

Treatment

- Acetaminophen for pain or fever.
- Symptomatic relief of allergy, upper respiratory infection, or other complaints.

Parent Call-back Is Needed for

- Persistent, changing, worsening, anxiety-provoking, or specific symptoms as outlined above.

Discussion

Headaches during childhood are common and only infrequently associated with serious underlying illness. The nonspecific nature of the symptom and the extensive differential diagnosis makes a thorough history and physical examination necessary for proper evaluation. There should be special concern when recurrent headache pain interferes with the patient's usual activities, is associated with other CNS symptoms, or frequently occurs in the early morning.

- *Acute illness* is responsible for most simple headaches, especially when *fever* is present. Headache usually disappears as the child becomes afebrile.
- *CNS infection* should be suspected when the child is febrile and appears lethargic or very irritable.
- *Head trauma* prior to the onset of severe headache suggests the possibility of a concussion or CNS bleed. Evaluation is needed when other CNS symptoms are present.
- *Sinusitis* or sinus congestion is suggested by associated rhinitis, especially when it is purulent. The headache may be localized over the region of one or more sinuses. (The frontal sinuses develop after age 6 years, but others are present earlier.)
- *Allergic rhinitis* may cause headache associated with sneezing, red or itching eyes, and a known history of allergy.
- *Migraine* or *vascular headaches* may be uni- or bilateral, preceded by an aura, and relieved after sleeping or vomiting. They often follow stressful situations and commonly occur as the child returns home from school. Early childhood migraine may have atypical presentation but may still be debilitating. A history of motion sickness or other family members with migraine makes this diagnosis more likely.
- *Tension-induced headaches* are often most severe toward the back of the head and tend to occur during or before a stressful episode.
- *Headaches caused by brain tumors* are most often worse early in the morning; hypoventilation and hypercapnia during sleep increase intracranial pressure. These headaches can be associated with vomiting and minimal nausea. Brain tumor is one of the least common causes of childhood headaches, but concern about this possibility is often the specific reason for the parent's call. When headaches sound benign, stress the need for a complete examination, but advise parents that these headaches do not sound as if they are being caused by a serious condition.

CLINICAL TIP. *Eye strain* is mentioned because it does *not* usually cause headache. It may, however, cause eye pain or discomfort late in the day.

General Principles

Common Symptoms

Emergencies and Traumas

Minor Infections

Infectious Diseases

Parenting Concerns

Infant Care

General
Principles

Common
Symptoms

Emergencies
and Traumas

Minor
Infections

Infectious
Diseases

Parenting
Concerns

Infant
Care

Pain on Urination (Dysuria)

Screening Questions

Background
- Name, age, sex?
- Chronic illness?
- Current medications and treatments?

Age
- How old is your child?

Pain
- Is pain severe or mild?
- Does the child have difficulty passing urine?
- Does pain occur each time the child urinates or only occasionally?

Duration
- When did symptoms first appear?

Bloody Urine
- Does the urine appear to contain blood?
- If yes, how often has that happened?

Fever
- If fever is present, when did it begin and how long has it been present?

Other Symptoms
- Does the child have diarrhea or other symptoms?
- Is there local skin irritation at the tip of the penis or around the vagina?

General Appearance
- Does the child look especially sick?

Jeffrey L. Brown: *Pediatric Telephone Medicine: Principles, Triage, and Advice,*
Second Edition. Copyright © 1994 J. B. Lippincott Company

119

Examine Immediately If

- The child appears toxic.
- Temperature is greater than 104°F (40°C).

Examine in the Near Future If

- There is frequent voiding (more often than once every 2 hours).
- Pain on urination occurs most times that the child urinates.
- Urine appears to contain blood.
- Local penile or vaginal irritation does not respond to symptomatic treatment.

See Related Sections

The toxic child (p. 61), fever (p. 53), and vaginitis (p. 195).

Treatment

- *Local irritation* of the genitalia can be treated with exposure to air and use of a protective ointment such as zinc oxide or steroid cream.
- *Difficulty passing urine* can be treated by sitting the child in a bathtub filled with lukewarm water and having the child urinate directly into the water.

Parent Call-back Is Needed for

- Persistent, changing, worsening, anxiety-provoking, or specific symptoms as outlined above.

Discussion

- *Local genital irritation* may be more common than infection as a cause of pain while urinating. Even if symptoms disappear quickly after local treatment, a urine culture should still be obtained at a later time. During active perineal irritation the culture may be less reliable, and bladder aspiration or catheterization may be necessary. Avoid these procedures unless symptoms are severe enough to require immediate use of systemic antibiotics.

120

- *Upper urinary tract infection* is suggested when fever and signs of toxicity are also present.
- *Lower urinary symptoms* are suggested by frequent urination and pain while voiding.
- *Urethral meatal irritation* or *narrowing* should be suspected when there is blood toward the end of passing urine or when the child must strain to urinate. Straining to pass urine may also be simply pain-related.
- *Gross hematuria* always requires examination.

CLINICAL TIP. Parents should collect a urine specimen from older children at home *before* coming to the office for evaluation. A jar *and its lid* should be boiled for 20 minutes and sealed until collection can be made. Genitalia should be gently washed with soap and water prior to urinating, and the collected specimen should be refrigerated until it is examined. If the child is unable to void at the time of examination, this home specimen is a next-best substitute.

General Principles

Common Symptoms

Emergencies and Traumas

Minor Infections

Infectious Diseases

Parenting Concerns

Infant Care

General
Principles

Common
Symptoms

Emergencies
and Traumas

Minor
Infections

Infectious
Diseases

Parenting
Concerns

Infant
Care

Skin Rashes (Dermatitis, Exanthems)

Screening Questions

Background
- Name, age, sex?
- Chronic illness?
- Current medications and treatments?
- Recent immunizations?

Location
- Where is the rash?
- Is it localized to one place, or does it cover the entire body?

Duration
- When did the rash first break out?

Itching
- Does the rash itch?

Appearance
- How would you describe the rash?
- Does it look like hives, welts, or bites?
- Are there blisters, whiteheads, or pimples?
- Is it flat, raised, or rough?
- Does it form circles with clear centers?
- Is the skin weeping or oozing?
- Is it diffuse like a sunburn or blotchy like measles?
- Does there seem to be bleeding or bruised areas under the skin?
- Are there any other symptoms such as sore throat, cold, vomiting, or diarrhea?

Contacts
- Has the child had recent exposure to others with a similar condition?

General Appearance
- Does the child look especially sick or have fever?

Jeffrey L. Brown: *Pediatric Telephone Medicine: Principles, Triage, and Advice,* Second Edition. Copyright © 1994 J. B. Lippincott Company

General Principles

Common Symptoms

Emergencies and Traumas

Minor Infections

Infectious Diseases

Parenting Concerns

Infant Care

Examine Immediately If

- The child appears toxic.
- There is extreme discomfort.
- The rash has a hemorrhagic quality, *i.e.,* it looks like bruising or bleeding under the skin.
- There is extreme parental anxiety.

Examine in the Near Future If

- Symptoms do not improve after treatment.
- Confirmation of diagnosis is needed.
- Symptoms suggest infection or other generalized illness.

See Related Sections

The toxic child (p. 61), insect bites (p. 151), athlete's foot (p. 177), chickenpox (p. 203), scarlet fever (p. 229).

Treatment

- *Itching.* Discontinue medications, especially antibiotics if they are currently being taken, and give antihistamines by mouth. Consider steroid cream for localized lesions when infection is not suspected.
- *Weeping lesions.* Use lukewarm water compresses.
- *Localized lesions* with blood-crusts, or pustules, or those that look infected. Use over-the-counter topical antibiotic creams to decrease contagion or prescription antibiotic creams for treatment.
- *Viral-appearing rashes* (blotchy or measles-like). Avoid contact with others until the child is examined. Use symptomatic treatment of other complaints. Advise pregnant contacts that the child has a viral rash.
- *Insect bites.* Use topical application of underarm deodorant containing aluminum salts or an astringent to decrease itching and local application of ice and oral antihistamines to decrease swelling.
- *Hives (urticaria).* Itching and swelling may be treated with oral antihistamines. If antibiotics or other medications are being taken, consider discontinuing them until the possibility of a *drug reaction* is resolved.
- *Contact dermatitis,* including *poison ivy.* Administer antihista-

124

mines by mouth. Wash area thoroughly with warm soapy water to remove plant oil from the skin. Steroid creams may be applied locally. Extensive exposure requires oral steroids after absence of infection and confirmation of diagnosis is made.

- *Fungal infections (athlete's foot and ringworm).* Use topical application of antifungal medicines. Compresses or soaks may be used for weeping areas. If the scalp is affected, oral medicines are usually needed.
- *Diaper dermatitis.* Use air exposure when practical and protective ointments when the diaper is worn.

CLINICAL TIP. Air exposure can be facilitated by cutting the elastic from the legs of disposable diapers or by pinning the front and back of the diaper to the baby's shirt with the diaper sides open. Protective zinc oxide ointment can be applied between diaper changes; it wipes off easily with baby oil. Diaper rash that looks like burned skin is probably infected with *Monilia* and may respond to over-the-counter antifungal creams.

Parent Call-back Is Needed for

- Persistent, changing, worsening, anxiety-provoking, or specific symptoms as outlined above.

Discussion

Telephone diagnosis and treatment of rashes can never substitute for in-person examination. However, accurate diagnosis is not always the goal of initial telephone contact: The primary objective is to give practical advice with regard to contagion, relief of symptoms, and potential dangers of illness. When rashes are associated with systemic disease, triage will depend on the severity of associated symptoms. The most common rashes are described below.

  ■ *Viral exanthems* are suggested by a generalized eruption consisting of multiple flat or slightly raised lesions that do not itch or have only minimal itching. The specific virus is not usually important unless the child has had recent contact with a pregnant woman. Exposure to a person with an upper respiratory tract infection, diarrhea, or vomiting makes ECHO or coxsackievirus infection more likely. High fever, cough, upper respiratory infection, and red eyes present before a rash appears suggest measles.

General
Principles

Common
Symptoms

Emergencies
and Traumas

Minor
Infections

Infectious
Diseases

Parenting
Concerns

Infant
Care

A young child with a 3-day history of high fever who develops a generalized rash coincidental with disappearance of fever suggests a diagnosis of roseola. Viral exanthems can occasionally be seen a few days to a week after administration of measles-mumps-rubella vaccine; they are not contagious and require no treatment.

- *Chickenpox (varicella)* usually presents as itchy blisters on a red base. Most often, the blisters begin on the chest, back, and abdomen and later spread to the face and extremities. See chickenpox (p. 203). Treatment is symptomatic, and the child should be isolated from others who have not had previous infection or vaccination. Some physicians request immediate examination to confirm diagnosis so that treatment with acyclovir can be started within 24 hours of rash onset.

- *Scarlet fever (scarlatina)* is suggested by a coarse, generalized sunburn-like rash most prominent in the groin and under the arms. It is usually associated with fever, vomiting, sore throat, and swollen lymph glands in the neck. A child with these symptoms should receive prompt medical attention. Many children with scarletina have only mild illness. Other less common but more serious illnesses that can be associated with a rash and symptoms similar to scarlet fever include *Kawasaki disease* and *staphylococcal* and *streptococcal toxic shock syndromes.*

- *Impetigo* may present as localized areas of pustules (white heads) with occasional vesicles (blisters), blood-crusts (scabs), and weeping areas. It may sometimes be described as looking like a cigarette burn. This should be treated with prescription antibiotics taken by mouth or applied topically. Application of over-the-counter topical antibiotic creams may be useful to decrease contagion.

- *Hives (urticaria)* can result from any potential allergen. When a new or unusual food has recently been added to the child's diet or when new medicines are being taken, they may provide a clue as to etiology. An extensive history is usually not fruitful or necessary unless hives are recurrent or associated with signs of generalized illness.

- *Hemorrhagic rashes* are commonly described as looking like "bleeding under the skin." All such rashes require immediate evaluation, especially when the child looks ill or has fever. These lesions can be caused by vasculitis as occurs with Henoch-Schönlein purpura, by problems of coagulation as occurs with idiopathic thrombocytopenic purpura or leukemia, or from generalized sepsis as might occur with meningococcemia or *Haemophilus influenzae* B infection.

- Circular (Annular) Lesions
  - *Erythema multiforme* is a variant of hives and presents as raised

126

circular lesions with relatively clear centers (target lesions). They are often itchy and may sometimes have a hemorrhagic quality. They frequently appear, disappear, and migrate at irregular intervals. When associated with a viral infection, lesions often coincide with other viral symptoms over 7 to 10 days. Antihistamines and steroids are often ineffective at controlling itching or swelling but may be useful as sedatives. Lesions caused by antibiotics and those caused by illness may be impossible to differentiate. Progression to serious allergic symptoms is uncommon.

- *Ringworm (tinea circinata)* is a fungal infection of the skin that may be described as an itchy patch of rough or scaly skin. The infected area develops central clearing as it increases in size.

- *Erythema chronicum migrans (ECM)* is a spreading circular rash that usually has little or no itching; borders can be slightly raised. Suspect this diagnosis when the patient lives in an area endemic to *Lyme disease,* if the rash occurs following a tick bite, or if there are also flu-like symptoms (headache, muscle aches, or low-grade fever) or joint pain. All patients with suspected ECM should be evaluated. Many experts recommend systemic antibiotic treatment for all patients with ECM regardless of serologic test results because of possible arthritic or neurological complications.

- *Eczema* (and/or *seborrhea*) is an irritation of the skin that almost always itches. Eczemoid areas may be rough or weeping and can occur on any body part. They are usually most prominent in the creases of the elbow, behind the knees, and behind the ears. Basic treatment includes infrequent bathing to avoid drying the skin; avoidance of wool clothing, blankets, carpets, and upholstery; application of steroid creams in the absence of infection; and oral antihistamines to control itching and for sedation.

- *Contact dermatitis* (including *poison ivy*) may be described as exposed areas of skin that are red, irritated, have blisters, or may be weeping. A straight line of itchy small blisters suggests poison ivy dermatitis. Oral antihistamines should be used for itching, wet compresses with plain water or Burrow's solution should be placed on weeping lesions, and calamine lotion may be applied to the others. Steroid creams or lotions may also be prescribed. For extreme discomfort or swelling, especially about the face, oral steroids are appropriate but should not be prescribed over the telephone. Both oral and topical steroids can worsen secondary bacterial infection when it is present.

- *Heat rash (miliaria)* is usually most prominent on the chest and upper back but may be generalized. It is often described as pimply but may also present as rough, red skin with tiny blisters (smaller than pinhead size). It can be as frequent in winter as in summer

General
Principles

Common
Symptoms

Emergencies
and Traumas

Minor
Infections

Infectious
Diseases

Parenting
Concerns

Infant
Care

because of overdressing. Heat rash can also be seen in association with febrile illnesses. Treatment consists of dressing the child in loose-fitting, lightweight cotton clothing to absorb perspiration. Affected areas should be powdered with cornstarch. Talcum powder may be used as a substitute but is more abrasive and less absorbent.

Notes

Notes

General
Principles

Common
Symptoms

Emergencies
and Traumas

Minor
Infections

Infectious
Diseases

Parenting
Concerns

Infant
Care

General
Principles

Common
Symptoms

Emergencies
and Traumas

Minor
Infections

Infectious
Diseases

Parenting
Concerns

Infant
Care

Notes

Trauma and Other Emergency Problems

General
Principles

Common
Symptoms

**Emergencies
and Traumas**

Minor
Infections

Infectious
Diseases

Parenting
Concerns

Infant
Care

Trauma
Basic Principles for Treating
 Trauma
Strains and Sprains
Fall from a Height
Trauma to the Head
Trauma to the Nose
Trauma to the Eye
Cuts (Lacerations)
Puncture Wounds

Other Emergencies
Insect Bites and Stings
Animal Bites
Human Bites
Nose Bleeds
Burns
Sunburn
Convulsions
Ingestion of Foreign Bodies
Poisonings and Ingestions

Basic Principles for Treating Trauma

- Immobilize the injured body part until it can be evaluated. Use a splint, sling, or pillow. See athletic injuries (p. 137).
- If bleeding is present, apply pressure directly over the bleeding area until it stops. A tourniquet is rarely needed.
- Apply ice or cool compresses when allowed by the child to decrease swelling.
- Elevate the injured part to decrease swelling.
- Apply heat after 2 days to increase blood supply and promote healing.

After an accident, parents should always be instructed to drive slowly and carefully or to obtain alternate transportation when bringing their child to a medical facility for evaluation.

General
Principles

Common
Symptoms

Emergencies
and Traumas

Minor
Infections

Infectious
Diseases

Parenting
Concerns

Infant
Care

Sprains and Strains (Athletic Injuries)

Screening Questions

Background
- Name, age, sex?
- Circumstances of the incident?
- General condition?

Examine Immediately for

- Extreme pain.
- Obvious bony deformity.

Examine Later for

- Pain, swelling, localized tenderness, or limitation of motion lasting longer than 24 hours.

Treatment

- Ice, elevation, and immobilization.
- Oral pain medication if needed.

Parent Call-back Is Needed for

- Persistent, changing, worsening, anxiety-provoking, or specific symptoms as outlined above.

Discussion

If the child is uncooperative and refuses to keep the extremity immobile, early examination is recommended.

Jeffrey L. Brown: *Pediatric Telephone Medicine: Principles, Triage, and Advice,*
Second Edition. Copyright © 1994 J. B. Lippincott Company

137

General Principles

Common Symptoms

Emergencies and Traumas

Minor Infections

Infectious Diseases

Parenting Concerns

Infant Care

CLINICAL TIPS

- When *ice* is applied to decrease swelling, the towel or cloth covering the ice pack should be wet to avoid insulating the cold-pack from the injured body part.
- A simple *arm sling* can be made by pinning the sleeve of the child's shirt to the body of the shirt at both elbow and wrist.
- A temporary *arm splint* for a small child can be constructed by folding a small magazine in half the long way and securing it to the arm with two handkerchiefs.
- A temporary *leg splint* for a small child can be fashioned from a pillow secured to the leg with two belts.
- A temporary *finger splint* can be made from a folded piece of cardboard and secured with two bandaids.
- A *toe splint* can be made by taping the injured toe to an adjacent toe with a bandaid.

General
Principles

Common
Symptoms

Emergencies
and Traumas

Minor
Infections

Infectious
Diseases

Parenting
Concerns

Infant
Care

Fall from a Height

Screening Questions

Background
- Name, age, sex?
- Circumstances of the incident?
- General condition?

Examine Immediately for

- Generalized ill appearance.
- Neurological signs, including altered state of consciousness, disorientation, incoordination, persistent vomiting, weakness, abnormal gait, slurred speech, or severe headache. See head trauma (p. 141).
- Bleeding from an ear or bruising behind the ear.
- Inability to move extremities symmetrically.
- Tender localized swelling of an extremity or body part.
- Severe pain.
- Extreme parental anxiety.

Parent Call-back Is Needed for

- Persistent, changing, worsening, anxiety-provoking, or specific symptoms as outlined above.

Discussion

When none of the signs described above are present, immediate examination is usually not necessary. However, if symptoms develop later or if the parent feels apprehensive about the accident or the child's appearance,

Jeffrey L. Brown: *Pediatric Telephone Medicine: Principles, Triage, and Advice,* Second Edition. Copyright © 1994 J. B. Lippincott Company

139

General
Principles

Common
Symptoms

Emergencies
and Traumas

Minor
Infections

Infectious
Diseases

Parenting
Concerns

Infant
Care

offer to evaluate the child. Parental anxiety can be disproportionately greater than expected for the degree of trauma when they experience guilt in addition to worry. When it is practical, parents should be instructed to completely undress the child to look for signs of redness, bruising, and swelling.

General
Principles

Common
Symptoms

Emergencies
and Traumas

Minor
Infections

Infectious
Diseases

Parenting
Concerns

Infant
Care

Trauma to the Head

Screening Questions

Background
- Name, age, sex?
- Circumstances of the incident?
- General condition?

Examine Immediately for

- Altered state of consciousness.
- Persistent vomiting.
- Lethargy lasting longer than 30 minutes.
- Other neurological signs, including severe and persistent headache, confusion, weakness, incoordination, abnormal gait, or slurred speech.
- Blood coming from an ear or bruising behind the ear.
- A history of loss of consciousness lasting longer than 1 minute.

Parent Call-back Is Needed for

- Persistent, changing, worsening, anxiety-provoking, or specific symptoms as outlined above.

Discussion

Children may act sleepy following a head injury, especially when the accident occurs late in the day or when there has been prolonged crying. They may also vomit once or twice because of excitation or an "adrenalin rush."

Jeffrey L. Brown: *Pediatric Telephone Medicine: Principles, Triage, and Advice,*
Second Edition. Copyright © 1994 J. B. Lippincott Company

General Principles

Common Symptoms

Emergencies and Traumas

Minor Infections

Infectious Diseases

Parenting Concerns

Infant Care

CLINICAL TIP. Neurological evaluation can sometimes be facilitated by *allowing children to sleep* following the injury and then arousing them at 1- to 2-hour intervals. It is a common parental misconception that keeping the child awake will prevent a *concussion.* If they vomit more than twice, are difficult to arouse, show signs of confused thinking, or have other neurological signs, they should be examined immediately.

Instant swelling over the forehead after trauma commonly results from bleeding under the skin and is a common cause for parental alarm. Children without other symptoms do not require further evaluation. A black-and-blue mark may last 1 week or longer. Black eyes appearing the next day are the result of blood drifting downward under the skin. Ice should be applied to the swelling if this is allowed by the child.

Soft spongy swelling anywhere over the skull of children less than 12 months old that lasts longer than 12 hours suggests the presence of a *skull fracture.* When swelling persists, the patient should be examined even when there are no symptoms.

Parents can be reassured that X-ray films of the skull or computerized axial tomographic (CAT) scan of the head are not usually necessary if the neurological examination is normal and the history sounds inconsistent with significant trauma; a nondisplaced skull fracture alone does not generally affect either the patient's treatment or the clinical course.

Trauma to the Nose

Screening Questions

Background
- Name, age, sex?
- Circumstances of the incident?
- General condition?

Examine Immediately for

- Extreme pain.
- Obvious bony deformity.
- Bleeding lasting longer than 20 minutes.

Examine Later for

- Persistent nasal swelling or difficulty breathing through one or both nostrils.

Treatment

- Stop bleeding by pressing both nostrils together while the patient is in a sitting or semisitting position.
- Apply ice or a cold compress to the swelling once bleeding has stopped.
- Administer pain-relieving medicines if needed.

Parent Call-back Is Needed for

- Persistent, changing, worsening, anxiety-provoking, or specific symptoms as outlined above.

Jeffrey L. Brown: *Pediatric Telephone Medicine: Principles, Triage, and Advice,*
Second Edition. Copyright © 1994 J. B. Lippincott Company

143

General Principles

Common Symptoms

Emergencies and Traumas

Minor Infections

Infectious Diseases

Parenting Concerns

Infant Care

Discussion

The youngster should be talked to in a quiet, reassuring tone since crying will increase blood supply to the face and increase bleeding. X-ray films taken when the child is less than 2 years old may not be helpful since little bone is present and cartilage will not show on the film. Persistent nasal swelling requires evaluation but not necessarily on an urgent basis: Many surgeons prefer to correct nasal fractures 2 or 3 weeks later, after swelling has decreased.

Trauma to the Eye

Screening Questions

Background
- Name, age, sex?
- Circumstances of the incident?
- General condition?

Examine Immediately for

- Persistent redness or tearing.
- Severe pain lasting longer than 30 minutes.
- Unequal pupils.
- Penetrating injuries.

Treatment

- Irrigate the eye with copious amounts of water if a foreign body is suspected or if a toxic substance has entered the eye.
- Apply ice to decrease swelling.
- Give oral analgesics for pain if needed.

Parent Call-back Is Needed for

- Persistent, changing, worsening, anxiety-provoking, or specific symptoms as outlined above.

Discussion

There are few instances when significant eye trauma does not cause pain, swelling, redness, or tearing. Allowing $\frac{1}{2}$ hour to see if symptoms disappear after injury screens out most minor problems. Prompt irrigation of

Jeffrey L. Brown: *Pediatric Telephone Medicine: Principles, Triage, and Advice,*
Second Edition. Copyright © 1994 J. B. Lippincott Company

General Principles

Common Symptoms

Emergencies and Traumas

Minor Infections

Infectious Diseases

Parenting Concerns

Infant Care

the eye with copious amounts of water is helpful for removing some foreign bodies and most toxic substances.

> **CLINICAL TIP.** Have the child lie on her back and pour room-temperature water from a drinking glass directly into the eye while holding the lids open with two fingers.

Cuts (Lacerations)

Screening Questions

Background
- Name, age, sex?
- Circumstances of the incident?
- General condition?

Examine Immediately for

- A gaping laceration that is longer than $\frac{1}{4}$ inch.
- Persistent bleeding.
- Persistent pain.
- Lacerations that may affect nerves or tendons.

Treatment

- Apply pressure directly over the wound until bleeding stops.
- Wash thoroughly with warm soap and water.
- Cover with a clean dressing.
- Refer for tetanus toxoid if indicated.
- Administration of analgesic medicine if needed.

Parent Call-back Is Needed for

- Persistent, changing, worsening, anxiety-provoking, or specific symptoms as outlined above.

Discussion

Lacerations about the head, face, and mouth may bleed more than expected from the size of the wound. Frantic trips to an emergency room

Jeffrey L. Brown: *Pediatric Telephone Medicine: Principles, Triage, and Advice,* Second Edition. Copyright © 1994 J. B. Lippincott Company

General
Principles

Common
Symptoms

Emergencies
and Traumas

Minor
Infections

Infectious
Diseases

Parenting
Concerns

Infant
Care

for a trivial injury can be avoided by having the parent apply pressure over the wound until bleeding stops and the size of the laceration can be evaluated. Sutures are usually not necessary for lacerations within the mouth unless they are large and gaping. This area usually heals rapidly without treatment, and surgical closure may increase chances for infection.

Puncture Wounds

Screening Questions

Background
- Name, age, sex?
- Circumstances of the incident?
- General condition?

Examine Immediately for

- Wounds with a diameter greater than $\frac{1}{8}$ inch.
- Severe pain.

Examine Later for

- Increasing pain, redness, or swelling at the site of the wound.

Treatment

- Wash well with hot soapy water.
- Apply pressure directly over the wound until bleeding stops.
- Refer for tetanus toxoid if indicated.
- Consider oral antibiotic treatment.
- Administration of oral analgesics if necessary.

Parent Call-back Is Needed for

- Persistent, changing, worsening, anxiety-provoking, or specific symptoms as outlined above.

Jeffrey L. Brown: *Pediatric Telephone Medicine: Principles, Triage, and Advice,*
Second Edition. Copyright © 1994 J. B. Lippincott Company

149

General
Principles

Common
Symptoms

**Emergencies
and Traumas**

Minor
Infections

Infectious
Diseases

Parenting
Concerns

Infant
Care

Discussion

Because of difficulty cleaning these wounds, they may be susceptible to infection. Ensure adequate follow-up, especially when puncture wounds involve the hands or feet or occurred in an obviously contaminated environment.

Insect Bites and Stings

Screening Questions

Background

■ Name, age, sex?
■ Circumstances of the incident?
■ General condition?
■ Known allergies to insect stings?

Examine Immediately for

- Pale or sweaty appearance following a bite or sting.
- Wheezing or difficulty breathing.
- Extreme swelling, pain, or itching at a site *different from* the bite or sting.

Examine Later for

- Persistent discomfort or swelling.
- Development of symptoms following tick bite: Signs of Lyme disease may include rash, fever, headache, or joint pain.

Treatment

- Apply ice and give antihistamine and analgesics for itching, swelling, or pain if necessary.
- Use topical application of aluminum salts (present in underarm deodorants) or astringents to decrease itching.

Jeffrey L. Brown: *Pediatric Telephone Medicine: Principles, Triage, and Advice*,
Second Edition. Copyright © 1994 J. B. Lippincott Company

Minor
Infections

Infectious
Diseases

Parenting
Concerns

Infant
Care

CLINICAL TIP. For tick removal, grasp the tick firmly with tweezers as close to the skin as possible. Pull straight out with gentle, steady pressure. Do not apply heat, cold, or chemical substances to the tick prior to its removal.

Discussion

When one considers the large numbers of individuals stung by hornets, wasps, and bees, serious allergic reactions are relatively uncommon. Those few reactions that are life-threatening obviously require immediate attention. The affected individual should be brought to an emergency room as quickly as possible. Patients can be instructed to take antihistamines and/or steroids if these are available before traveling to the hospital. Those with a known allergy to insect stings should carry a self-injecting epinephrine syringe.

Swelling following insect bites or stings is most severe in younger children. A simple mosquito bite can cause a small child's eye to become swollen closed. Red streaking along the path of lymphatics may follow a bite or sting and is more commonly caused by foreign protein in the lymphatics than by bacterial infection.

Tick bites may cause local irritation at the site of the bite. Suspect *Lyme disease* if it is prevalent in your area, when the child later develops viral-like symptoms, arthralgia, rash, or erythema chronicum migrans (a circular red rash with clearing at the center). See p. 217.

General
Principles

Common
Symptoms

Emergencies
and Traumas

Minor
Infections

Infectious
Diseases

Parenting
Concerns

Infant
Care

Animal Bites

Screening Questions

Background
- Name, age, sex?
- Circumstances of the incident?
- General condition?

Examine Immediately for

- Lacerations longer than $\frac{1}{4}$ inch.
- Persistent bleeding.
- *Unprovoked* bites of domestic or wild animals but especially dogs, bats, skunks, raccoons, foxes, or monkeys.

Examine Later for

- Increasing redness, pain, or swelling at the wound site.
- A bite by an apparently healthy or friendly domestic animal that cannot be located or that has not been immunized against rabies.
- Minimal injury that occurred during undocumented circumstances.

Treatment

- Wash the wound immediately with copious amounts of warm soapy water.
- Apply pressure directly over the wound site to stop bleeding.
- Apply ice to decrease swelling.
- Give oral analgesics for pain if necessary.
- Refer for tetanus toxoid if indicated.
- Refer for rabies treatment if indicated.
- Notify local police to ensure adequate follow-up of the animal.

Jeffrey L. Brown: *Pediatric Telephone Medicine: Principles, Triage, and Advice,* Second Edition. Copyright © 1994 J. B. Lippincott Company

153

Minor
Infections

Infectious
Diseases

Parenting
Concerns

Infant
Care

Parent Call-back Is Needed for

- Persistent, changing, worsening, anxiety-provoking, or specific symptoms as outlined above.

Discussion

An accurate history is essential to determine the *risk of rabies.* Bites occurring while the child is playing with, teasing, or feeding a well-appearing animal carry little potential risk. Rabies is even less likely when a domestic animal is known to be immunized. Bites from small rodents (mice, rats, and squirrels) are not considered dangerous. When you are uncertain about the prevalence of rabies in your area, information can usually be obtained by contacting the local Board of Health.

Despite the social problems that may result, parents should notify the police even when their child has been bitten by a neighbor's pet. Such action may be helpful for establishing blame if medical complications occur later. Also, the report helps to assure medical follow-up of the animal and documentation if it has a tendency to bite others.

Puncture *wounds of the hand,* especially from *cat bites,* are at risk for developing severe infections, and some physicians routinely prescribe prophylactic antibiotics.

Human Bites

Screening Questions

Background
- Name, age, sex?
- Circumstances of the incident?
- General condition?

Examine Immediately for

- Laceration larger than $\frac{1}{4}$ inch.
- Persistent pain or bleeding.

Examine Later for

- Increasing redness, swelling, or pain at the wound site.

Treatment

- Wash the wound vigorously with copious amounts of warm soapy water.
- Apply pressure directly over the wound to stop bleeding.
- Apply ice to minimize discomfort and swelling.
- Give oral analgesics for pain if necessary.
- Refer for administration of tetanus toxoid if indicated.

Parent Call-back Is Needed for

- Persistent, changing, worsening, anxiety-provoking, or specific symptoms as outlined above.

General
Principles

Common
Symptoms

Emergencies
and Traumas

Minor
Infections

Infectious
Diseases

Parenting
Concerns

Infant
Care

Discussion

The primary morbidity from human bites is most often pain and mental anguish. Local wound care is usually adequate for good management. However, some practitioners routinely prescribe prophylactic antibiotics after human bites, especially when significant puncture wounds or lacerations are present.

Nose Bleeds (Epistaxis)

Screening Questions

Background
- Name, age, sex?
- Circumstances of the incident?
- General condition?
- Other similar episodes?
- Current illness, medications, or treatments?

Examine Immediately for

- Bleeding lasting longer than 30 minutes.

Examine Later for

- Recurrent bleeding from the same nostril.
- Persistent bleeding following trauma.

Treatment

- Semisitting position.
- Reassurance until the child stops crying.
- Pressure to compress the lower portion of the bleeding nostril(s).
- Vaporizer for the sleeping child.

Parent Call-back Is Needed for

- Persistent, changing, worsening, anxiety-provoking, or specific symptoms as outlined above.

Jeffrey L. Brown: *Pediatric Telephone Medicine: Principles, Triage, and Advice,*
Second Edition. Copyright © 1994 J. B. Lippincott Company

General
Principles

Common
Symptoms

Emergencies
and Traumas

Minor
Infections

Infectious
Diseases

Parenting
Concerns

Infant
Care

Discussion

Control of *apprehension* is important because crying increases facial blood supply and worsens the bleeding. Embarrassment may occur when a child bleeds in the presence of peers, so reassurance and support are especially important.

Evening nose bleeds are common during winter months from breathing dry heated air; vaporizers or humidifiers may be helpful. Epistaxis secondary to irritation from an *upper respiratory tract infection* or *allergic rhinitis* may be prevented by treating the underlying conditions.

CLINICAL TIP. Errors made when treating nose bleeds include pinching the nostrils for too short a period of time and pressing on the bridge of the nose rather than the lower part of the nostril. Most bleeding comes from vessels along the lower portion of the septum, and pressure applied elsewhere is of little or no value. Ice packs are usually of little help.

Recurrent bleeding from the same nostril suggests a superficial blood vessel that will respond to cauterization. One would expect that if a nose bleed follows trauma, this information would be offered as part of the initial complaint. To the embarrassment of an unwary practitioner, this essential history may not be forthcoming unless a direct question is asked.

General
Principles

Common
Symptoms

Emergencies
and Traumas

Minor
Infections

Infectious
Diseases

Parenting
Concerns

Infant
Care

Burns

Screening Questions

Background
- Name, age, sex?
- Circumstances of the incident?
- General condition?

Examine Immediately for

- Any burned area larger than 3 inches in diameter.

Treatment

- Apply cool compresses immediately.
- Wash with lukewarm soapy water.
- Cover with a clean dressing (preferably a nonsticking pad).
- Give oral analgesics.

Parent Call-back Is Needed for

- Persistent, changing, worsening, anxiety-provoking, or specific symptoms.

Discussion

All large burns should be examined and dressed immediately. This may also be necessary for smaller burns in difficult-to-keep clean areas, such as the hands of small children. Cool water applied immediately to the burn stops skin from cooking after the heat source has been removed. Topical antibiotics are often prescribed. Some physicians recommend prophylactic oral antibiotics for moderate-sized second-degree burns to prevent secondary infection.

Jeffrey L. Brown: *Pediatric Telephone Medicine: Principles, Triage, and Advice,*
Second Edition. Copyright © 1994 J. B. Lippincott Company

Sunburn

Screening Questions

Background
■ Name, age, sex?
■ Circumstances of the incident?
■ General condition?

Examine Immediately for

• Temperature greater than 101°F (38.4°C).
• Toxic-appearing child. See the toxic child (p. 61).

Examine Later for

• Large areas of weeping or oozing skin.
• Persistent pain or discomfort after home treatment.

Treatment

• Analgesics for pain or itching.
• Antihistamines may be used for sedation.
• Cool compresses if skin is weeping or oozing.
• Elevation of affected extremities when practical.

Discussion

Few sunburns become true medical emergencies, but many can cause extreme discomfort. When sunburn affects large areas of the body, the child may develop chills, fever, lethargy, or loss of appetite.

Jeffrey L. Brown: *Pediatric Telephone Medicine: Principles, Triage, and Advice,*
Second Edition. Copyright © 1994 J. B. Lippincott Company

General
Principles

Common
Symptoms

Emergencies
and Traumas

Minor
Infections

Infectious
Diseases

Parenting
Concerns

Infant
Care

CLINICAL TIP. *Prevention of sunburn* is the most important element of sun care:

- Small children should *avoid* the sun whenever possible. When avoidance is not practical, sun-blocking agents should be used:
- These should be tested for skin sensitivity on a small portion of the child's body the day before general application is to be made.
- Use a protection number of at least 15 and protect against UVA and UVB rays.
- Apply blocks at least 20 minutes before going outside.
- Apply evenly and carefully to avoid "skip" areas.
- Reapply frequently, especially if the child is swimming.

Convulsions (Seizures)

Screening Questions

Background
- Name, age, sex?
- Fever?
- Recent illness or medication?
- Trauma, ingestion, or aspiration?
- Chronic medical conditions?
- Present condition?

Examine Immediately for

- All generalized convulsions unless there is a previous history of similar episodes.

Treatment

- Position the child to assure adequate airway.
- Use Heimlich maneuver if aspiration is suspected.
- Place the child on the floor near a telephone for observation while help is being called.
- Arrange transportation: Call police, ambulance, or a neighbor (whichever will respond first).

Discussion

Reassure parents that most convulsions are not life-threatening; even when there is transient breath-holding or change in color, most will stop spontaneously without treatment. The child should be placed on the floor near a phone to allow constant observation while advice is sought and

General
Principles

Common
Symptoms

Emergencies
and Traumas

Minor
Infections

Infectious
Diseases

Parenting
Concerns

Infant
Care

transportation arranged. Rapid transportation generally takes priority over obtaining an ambulance with emergency equipment. A parent should not drive alone, even after the seizure has stopped, because a recurrence while in transit could be dangerous, and because the parent is usually too nervous to drive safely.

Ingestion of Foreign Bodies

Screening Questions

Background
- Name, age, sex?
- Circumstances of the incident?
- General condition?

Examine Immediately for

- Cough lasting longer than 10 minutes.
- Wheezing or difficulty breathing.
- Persistent abdominal or chest pain.
- Persistent vomiting, drooling, or difficulty swallowing.
- Bloody stools.

X-ray Immediately for

- The above symptoms.
- Ingested objects with sharp or pointed edges.
- Ingested "button" batteries.

Parent Call-back Is Needed for

- Persistent, changing, worsening, anxiety-provoking, or specific symptoms as outlined above.

Discussion

The most commonly swallowed objects do not usually harm the child. When the object is small enough to pass easily through the esophagus and into the stomach, it will usually pass through the rectum within 24 to 48 hours. Coins, buttons, and marbles are common offenders. Some physi-

Minor
Infections

Infectious
Diseases

Parenting
Concerns

Infant
Care

cians X-ray all children who have swallowed coins and similar-shaped objects because of their potential to become trapped in the esophagus. Others X-ray only when the child is symptomatic while maintaining frequent telephone contact.

"Button batteries" can be corrosive to the intestine or esophagus, and their removal may be necessary. Plastic objects may not appear on X-ray films; glass objects may be seen if the glass contains lead. When X-rays are ordered, chest (including the neck), and abdominal films should be taken.

Poisonings and Ingestions

Screening Questions

Background

- Name, age, sex?
- Acute or chronic illnesses?
- Telephone number of caretaker?
- *Name and dose* of substance ingested?
- If a *prescription drug:*
  - Name of the pharmacy?
  - Pharmacy telephone number?
  - Prescription number?
- If a *nonprescription drug:*
  - Note contents, ingredients, and quantity.
- If a *liquid:*
  - Does the substance smell like a solvent (cleaning fluid, gasoline, turpentine, etc.)?
- *Quantity* consumed or amount remaining in the bottle?
- Amount of *time* since ingestion?
- *Symptoms* present?
  - Does the child have lethargy, nausea, vomiting, difficulty breathing, pain, or other symptoms?
  - General condition?

Examine Immediately for

- Callers not known to the examiner or those thought to be unreliable.
- Ingestion of a suspected central nervous system (CNS) depressant or other substance in quantities thought to be toxic.
- Ingestion of caustic substances.
- Significant symptoms following ingestion.

Instructions to Parents

- If small amounts of *solvent-containing substances* have been ingested, do not induce vomiting as this might cause aspiration

Jeffrey L. Brown: *Pediatric Telephone Medicine: Principles, Triage, and Advice,*
Second Edition. Copyright © 1994 J. B. Lippincott Company

167

General
Principles

Common
Symptoms

**Emergencies
and Traumas**

Minor
Infections

Infectious
Diseases

Parenting
Concerns

Infant
Care

pneumonia. The child should drink large amounts of liquids, and the parent should be instructed to watch for wheezing or cough that may develop up to 24 hours later.

- When a small amount of a substance with moderate toxicity has been ingested, induce *vomiting* as follows:
- Tell the caller to get a paper and pencil to write down instructions.
- Give the child large quantities of any fluid to drink.

CLINICAL TIP. If *syrup of ipecac* is not available in the home, take the child to the nearest pharmacy. Bring a tablespoon to administer 1 tablespoon (15 ml) of syrup of ipecac while at the pharmacy. Also bring a plastic bag to be used in case emesis occurs while on the way home. If no vomiting has occurred after 20 minutes, half that dose should be repeated. Continue offering clear liquids by mouth.

- When you are uncertain about the toxicity of the ingested substance, tell the parent you will call back with instructions within 5 minutes. Then call the local Poison Control Center for advice.

Poison control telephone number _____ .

Discussion

When there is a question about history reliability, it is safer to induce vomiting (unless the substance has the smell of a volatile hydrocarbon or the child is very lethargic) and to examine the child. Vomiting helps to protect the child when the parent underestimates the amount of the ingestion and may also provide a learning experience for both child and parent. Bringing a spoon with the child to the pharmacy saves travel time and halves waiting time before the ipecac can be administered. Since time of administration to time of emesis is usually 20 minutes, most children will not begin throwing up until after they return home. Taking a plastic bag in the car is worthwhile insurance, however. Some clinicians administer activated charcoal in addition to, or in place of, ipecac. When in doubt, discuss this issue with the local Poison Control Center.

Vomiting should not be induced in the presence of *volatile hydrocarbons*. In most cases, children will put a small amount of a substance to their lips and spill the rest on their clothing, giving the impression of a larger ingestion than actually took place. Parents should be alerted that respiratory symptoms may not occur until 12 to 24 hours following ingestion. X-ray films can be delayed since lung changes may not appear until later.

Ingestion of a *single tablet* of any adult medication may cause symptoms consistent with the action of the medicine but is rarely dangerous. *Poison Control Center numbers* are available in most cities. Use their help whenever you are uncertain about the toxicity or content of the substance ingested. Carry the number on your person for use when you are not in your office or at the hospital. It is preferred to have the practitioner call the Center and then call the patient back. When evaluation is necessary, you can then tell the parent the best location to administer treatment (home, office, or hospital).

Most Commonly Ingested Medications

Acetylsalicylic Acid (Aspirin)
The toxic dose is approximately 1 grain (65 mg) per 2 pounds of body weight. The initial sign of toxicity is often hyperventilation (rapid breathing). Signs of metabolic acidosis may occur later.

Acetaminophen (Liquiprin, Tylenol, Tempra, Datril)
The toxic dose is approximately 1 grain (65 mg) per 2 pounds of body weight. Symptoms do not usually appear immediately after overdose but may occur 2 to 3 days later. Central nervous system depression and liver dysfunction may result. Rapid treatment will decrease the likelihood of hepatic toxicity substantially.

"Cold" Preparations
These are usually not toxic unless taken in very large amounts. They may cause symptoms of irritability, lethargy, and occasional hypertension. No treatment is usually necessary.

Vitamins
Large amounts are not usually toxic as a single ingestion but can be extremely dangerous *when they contain iron.* X-ray films of the abdomen may confirm the number of tablets ingested because they may be visible on the film. Iron intoxication can cause rapid onset of severe illness, including shock. When ingestion of a moderate quantity of iron-containing tablets is suspected, immediate evaluation is indicated.

Birth Control Pills
These are not toxic, but withdrawal vaginal bleeding may occur in young females a few days after ingestion.

General
Principles

Common
Symptoms

Emergencies
and Traumas

Minor
Infections

Infectious
Diseases

Parenting
Concerns

Infant
Care

Tranquilizers

Single-tablet ingestions may result in lethargy or hyperactivity. Treatment is not necessary. When there is any question about the number of tablets ingested, patient evaluation is usually necessary.

Notes

General Principles

Common Symptoms

Emergencies and Traumas

Minor Infections

Infectious Diseases

Parenting Concerns

Infant Care

Notes

Notes

General Principles

Common Symptoms

Emergencies and Traumas

Minor Infections

Infectious Diseases

Parenting Concerns

Infant Care

173

General
Principles

Common
Symptoms

Emergencies
and Traumas

Minor
Infections

Infectious
Diseases

Parenting
Concerns

Infant
Care

Notes

Minor Localized Infections

General
Principles

Common
Symptoms

Emergencies
and Traumas

**Minor
Infections**

Infectious
Diseases

Parenting
Concerns

Infant
Care

Athlete's Foot
Canker Sores
Cold Sores
Head Lice
Pink Eye

Pinworm
Sty
Swimmer's Ear
Thrush
Vaginal Discharge

General
Principles

Common
Symptoms

Emergencies
and Traumas

Athlete's Foot (Tinea Pedis)

Screening Questions

Background
- Name, age, sex?
- Current illness, medication, treatment?
- Other symptoms?

Description

Athlete's foot is caused by a fungus infection of the skin between the toes. This may be described as fissuring, cracking, redness, itching, and pain. Sometimes small blisters or weeping skin are seen. When these symptoms are seen in prepubertal youngsters, eczema as well as athlete's foot should be suspected.

Contagion

Minimal. Shower slippers are recommended.

Treatment

- Expose feet to the air as frequently as possible.
- Apply topical antifungal agents.

Examination Needed for

- Confirmation of diagnosis.
- Symptoms persisting after 2 weeks of topical medication.
- Excessive redness, blistering, or pain suggestive of secondary bacterial infection.

General
Principles

Common
Symptoms

Emergencies
and Traumas

Canker Sores

Screening Questions

Background
- Name, age, sex?
- Current illness, medication, treatment?
- Other symptoms?

Description

Canker sores are single or multiple painful ulcerations of the mouth that can be caused by a variety of different agents. They may occur in association with stress or with illness and may be precipitated by minor trauma. They are often recurrent, and the etiology is undetermined. But lesions on the gums, especially when associated with fever or other systemic symptoms, suggest herpes simplex infection.

Contagion

Minimal unless herpes simplex is suspected.

Treatment

- Avoid foods that are spicy, salty, or contain citric acid (orange, lemon, grapefruit, etc.). These cause uncomfortable burning.
- After eating, rinse the mouth with a clear liquid to remove debris.
- Analgesics may be given for pain. Sedation with antihistamines may be desired, especially at nighttime. Avoid liquid medicines that contain alcohol since they may cause discomfort.
- Topical anaesthetic preparations may provide symptomatic relief.

Jeffrey L. Brown: *Pediatric Telephone Medicine: Principles, Triage, and Advice,*
Second Edition. Copyright © 1994 J. B. Lippincott Company

179

General
Principles

Common
Symptoms

Emergencies
and Traumas

**Minor
Infections**

Infectious
Diseases

Parenting
Concerns

Infant
Care

Examination Needed for

- Confirmation of diagnosis.
- Temperature higher than 101°F (38.4°C) and numerous mouth lesions.
- Other systemic symptoms.

General
Principles

Common
Symptoms

Emergencies
and Traumas

Cold Sores (Fever Blisters, Herpes Simplex Infection)

Screening Questions

Background
- Name, age, sex?
- Current illness, medication, treatment?
- Other symptoms?

Description

Cold sores are described as single or multiple blisters (vesicles) that are usually located near border of the lips. They may ooze serous fluid or develop crusting. They are often recurrent and persist for 7 to 10 days despite treatment. Lesions may appear in association with psychological or physical stress.

Contagion

Significant. Avoid skin-to-skin contact with others and use frequent hand washing.

Treatment

Sores may be treated with the application of topical astringents. Some physicians recommend use of topical acyclovir ointment. If secondary bacterial infection is suspected, topical or oral antibiotics may be prescribed.

Examination Needed for

- Confirmation of diagnosis; especially to rule out impetigo.
- Lesions persisting longer than 7 days.
- Spreading or worsening lesions.

General
Principles

Common
Symptoms

Emergencies
and Traumas

Head Lice (Pediculosis)

Screening Questions

Background
- Name, age, sex?
- Current illness, medication, treatment?
- Other symptoms?

Description

Pediculosis is an infestation of the scalp with lice. This may cause itching, rash, or swollen glands in the back of the neck. Lice can sometimes be seen, but more commonly the eggs or nits will be found approximately $\frac{1}{4}$ inch from the base of the hair shaft. They are most likely to be seen at the back of the neck or temples. Eggs are white, opaque, have a diameter of approximately $\frac{1}{16}$ inch, and are firmly attached to the hair shaft.

Contagion

Significant. Avoid head-to-head contact (playing, wrestling, etc.) and sharing of hats, combs, and other similar objects.

Treatment

- Application of *medicated shampoo* will kill the lice and most of the eggs. Depending on the product used, a second washing may be recommended. Individual eggs must be removed from the hair shaft with a fine-toothed comb or tweezers. Application of "nit-removing" lotions may be helpful to loosen adhesive that attaches eggs to the hairs. Reexamination should be scheduled to look for signs of reinfestation.
- *Linens,* towels, and clothing currently in use should be washed,

General
Principles

Common
Symptoms

Emergencies
and Traumas

**Minor
Infections**

Infectious
Diseases

Parenting
Concerns

Infant
Care

placed in the dryer, or ironed, with special attention given to seams. Any of these procedures will kill both eggs and lice.
- *Treatment of contacts.* No treatment of contacts is necessary unless signs of infestation are found.

Examination Needed for

- Confirmation of diagnosis.
- Secondary infection when believed to be present.

General
Principles

Common
Symptoms

Emergencies
and Traumas

Pink Eye (Conjunctivitis)

Screening Questions

Background
- Name, age, sex?
- Current illness, medication, treatment?
- Other symptoms?

Description

Conjunctivitis is described as a creamy or watery discharge coming from one or both eyes. Sometimes redness of the white part of the eye is present without discharge. Conjunctivitis may be caused by viral or bacterial infection or by chemical, mechanical, or allergic irritation. When purulent discharge is seen together with purulent rhinitis, an associated ear infection should be suspected in susceptible children.

Contagion

Significant. Preschoolers should avoid contact with other children when practical. Frequent hand washing and separate wash cloths and towels are recommended.

Treatment

- Nonpurulent conjunctivitis occurring in association with an upper respiratory tract infection is usually *viral* in etiology and may be treated by wiping away discharge with a moist cotton ball.
- When conjunctivitis is associated with eye itching, sneezing, or other *allergic* symptoms, it may be treated with oral antihistamines or instillation of anti-inflammatory drops.
- When purulent discharge is present and thought to be caused by *bacterial* infection, topical antibiotics are necessary. The following instructions should be given:

Jeffrey L. Brown: *Pediatric Telephone Medicine: Principles, Triage, and Advice,* Second Edition. Copyright © 1994 J. B. Lippincott Company

185

Ophthalmic antibiotic drops or ointment should be applied to
the inner portion of the lower eyelid three to four times a day for a
minimum of 3 days even when symptoms resolve more quickly.
Persons who instill the medication should wash their hands after treatment.

> **CLINICAL TIP.** When instillation of eyedrops is so difficult that it
> causes extreme parental anxiety and household turmoil, a short
> course of oral antibiotics can be an equally effective substitute.

Examination Needed for

- Presence of fever, systemic symptoms, or generalized rash.
- Confirmation of diagnosis.
- Symptoms lasting longer than 3 days or worsening after treat-
ment.
- Redness and swelling of the eyelids and/or the area around the
eye.
- Significant pain and tearing.
- Eye redness following trauma.

Discussion

Most conjunctival irritation reflects simple viral or bacterial infection and
will respond promptly to treatment. However, *other more serious conditions* requiring early examination that can cause a red eye include unnoticed trauma, presence of foreign body, and vasculitis associated with
staphylococcal, streptococcal, Kawasaki or collagen disease. Marked
swelling of the area around the eye or the presence of fever may also suggest *periorbital cellulitis* or *uveitis*.

See Related Sections

Trauma to the eye (p. 145), dermatitis (p. 123).

Pinworm (Oxyuriasis)

Screening Questions

Background
- Name, age, sex?
- Current illness, medication, treatment?
- Other symptoms?

Description

Pinworm is an infestation of the rectum and occasionally the vagina. Children frequently complain of itching and sometimes pain at these areas especially late at night and early in the morning. Heavy infestations occasionally cause abdominal pain. Intense itching may lead to scratching and local irritation of the rectum and genitalia. Worms are approximately $\frac{1}{4}$ inch long, white, and have the appearance of thick threads. Diagnosis is confirmed when live worms are seen at examination of the rectum or when microscopic eggs are located on a slide taken from the perirectal area.

> **CLINICAL TIP.** Parents should be told to avoid bathing the child before coming to the office for evaluation since this may remove evidence of infestation.

Contagion

Significant. Handwashing is recommended before eating or preparing food and after using the toilet. All household members require treatment.

General
Principles

Common
Symptoms

Emergencies
and Traumas

Minor
Infections

Infectious
Diseases

Parenting
Concerns

Infant
Care

Treatment

Oral prescription medications are given to all household contacts, even when they are asymptomatic. A second course of treatment 1 week later is usually recommended. After the medicine is taken, all linens, towels, bedclothes, and underwear in current use should be laundered. Special attention should be paid to items presently in the hamper, and hands should be washed after handling them. Strict hand washing should also be employed for the next few days before eating and after using the toilet.

Examination Needed for

- Confirmation of diagnosis.

General
Principles

Common
Symptoms

Emergencies
and Traumas

Minor
Infections

Infectious
Diseases

Parenting
Concerns

Infant
Care

Sty

Screening Questions

Background
- Name, age, sex?
- Current illness, medication, treatment?
- Other symptoms?

Description

A sty is a localized red swelling of either the upper or lower eyelid. It is sometimes tender or painful.

Contagion

Minimal.

Treatment

Because a sty is essentially a pimple of the eyelid, treatment should consist only of *warm water compresses* when they are allowed by the child. Antibiotic ointments are of limited or no value. Occasionally, systemic antibiotics are needed when there is surrounding inflammation.

Examination Needed for

- Confirmation of diagnosis.
- Significant pain, fever, or systemic symptoms.
- Increasing eyelid swelling or pain.

General
Principles

Common
Symptoms

Emergencies
and Traumas

Swimmer's Ear (External Otitis)

Screening Questions

Background
- Name, age, sex?
- Current illness, medication, treatment?
- Other symptoms?

Description

Swimmer's ear is suggested when the child has ear pain that is worsened by pressing on the area around the ear canal, especially the cartilaginous button (tragus) just in front on the ear. It is especially common during summer months. This condition is caused by skin irritation within the ear canal and does not affect the middle ear. Fever and respiratory infections commonly seen with middle ear infections are not usually associated with external otitis.

Contagion

None.

Treatment

- Avoid swimming or allowing water to enter the ear canal. A cotton plug coated with petroleum jelly will usually provide a waterproof seal during swimming or hair washing. Soft moldable plastic ear plugs may be effective.
- Analgesics for pain.
- Application of heat.
- Administration of ear drops containing acetic acid, cortisone, antibiotics, or a combination of these.

Jeffrey L. Brown: *Pediatric Telephone Medicine: Principles, Triage, and Advice,*
Second Edition. Copyright © 1994 J. B. Lippincott Company

Examination Needed for

- Confirmation of diagnosis.
- Worsening pain after 2 days of treatment.
- Ear discharge.
- Fever or other systemic symptoms.

Thrush (Oral Candidiasis)

Screening Questions

Background
- Name, age, sex?
- Current illness, medication, treatment?
- Other symptoms?

Description

Thrush is described as white plaques in the mouth (usually of infants) that are localized to the tongue, inner lips, or inner cheeks. They cannot be removed when wiped with a clean handkerchief. The infection is caused by a yeast called *Candida* or *Monilia*. Other symptoms are not usually present, but diaper rash can occur when this organism is passed along with stool into the diaper region.

Contagion

None.

Treatment

The specific treatment is topical application of a prescription antifungal agent. Swabbing infected areas with 1 percent gentian violet solution (available without prescription) four times daily after meals can be equally effective. Advise parents that gentian violet is messy and esthetically unpleasant. The label reads "Not for internal use," but this solution is safe when used as prescribed.

Examination Needed for

- Confirmation of diagnosis.
- Persistent infection after 7 days of treatment.

Jeffrey L. Brown: *Pediatric Telephone Medicine: Principles, Triage, and Advice,* Second Edition. Copyright © 1994 J. B. Lippincott Company

General
Principles

Common
Symptoms

Emergencies
and Traumas

**Minor
Infections**

Infectious
Diseases

Parenting
Concerns

Infant
Care

Vaginal Discharge (Vaginitis)

Screening Questions

Background
- Name, age, sex?
- Current illness, medication, treatment?
- Other symptoms?

Description

- Vaginal discharge and swollen genitalia in *infants* can be present during the first few days of life as a reflection of the mother's high estrogen levels. When hormone levels drop, the baby menstruates and a bloody vaginal discharge results. This condition is self-limited, and no treatment is necessary.
- Vaginal discharge in *preschool-* and *school-aged* children may be caused by
  - Improper wiping (back to front) of the rectal area that sweeps stool across the genitalia from the rectum.
  - Bubble bath or shampoo in bathwater entering the vagina and acting as a local irritant.
  - Wearing nonabsorbent nylon underwear or pantyhose that promotes poor hygiene.
  - Intentional or unintentional presence of a vaginal foreign body (*e.g.,* toilet paper) causing irritation and infection.
- Vaginal discharge in *teenagers* can be caused by the same agents seen in adults; thorough evaluation is indicated, especially when the patient is sexually active. Early postpubertal youngsters may complain of a hormone-induced *physiologic discharge* described as clear or slightly yellow and nonodorous; no treatment or evaluation is needed.
  - Vaginal infection, especially by *Monilia,* can follow *antibiotic use.* This can be seen at any age but is more common in postpubertal teenagers.
  - *Mechanical irritation* may lead to vaginal discharge and occasional infection at any age excluding infancy. This may occur

General
Principles

Common
Symptoms

Emergencies
and Traumas

Minor
Infections

Infectious
Diseases

Parenting
Concerns

Infant
Care

following manipulation during *masturbation* or as the result of *pinworm*.

Contagion

Depends on the offending organism.

Examination Needed for

- Discharge containing blood (except in infants) or pus.
- Discharge associated with foul odor.
- Discharge in sexually active patients.
- Significant vaginal, labial, or anal irritation unresponsive to changes in hygiene.
- Suspicion of foreign body.
- Suspicion of trauma or sexual abuse.
- Severe itching (especially at nighttime or early morning) suggesting pinworm.
- Need to distinguish between infection and physiologic discharge.
- Recurrent episodes.

Treatment

- Sitz baths, white cotton underpants, avoidance of bubble bath and shampoo in bathwater, and instructions concerning proper wiping.

> **CLINICAL TIP.** It is sometimes forgotten that shampoo contains ingredients identical to bubble bath. When children wash their hair while seated in the tub, perfumes and detergents in the shampoo can be an unsuspected cause of vaginitis or whole-body rash.

- Administration of intravaginal vinegar with a syringe may lower vaginal pH, but most children will not tolerate this treatment. One-half cup of vinegar added to a partially filled bathtub used as a sitz bath is a next-best alternative.
- A trial of antibiotics for nonspecific vaginitis in prepubertal girls is often successful even when cultures have been "negative."
- Discontinuation of antibiotics and administration of antifungal

agents may be tried for postpubertal girls. Regular dietary inclusion of yogurt containing live cultures of lactobacilli or lactobacillus-containing capsules may be useful for preventing recurrent monilial vaginitis.

- Application of cortisone creams to external genitalia may interrupt an itch–rub cycle once pinworm and other forms of irritation have been excluded.

General
Principles

Common
Symptoms

Emergencies
and Traumas

**Minor
Infections**

Infectious
Diseases

Parenting
Concerns

Infant
Care

General
Principles

Common
Symptoms

Emergencies
and Traumas

Minor
Infections

Infectious
Diseases

Parenting
Concerns

Infant
Care

Notes

Notes

General
Principles

Common
Symptoms

Emergencies
and Traumas

Minor
Infections

Infectious
Diseases

Parenting
Concerns

Infant
Care

General Principles

Common Symptoms

Emergencies and Traumas

Minor Infections

Infectious Diseases

Parenting Concerns

Infant Care

Notes

Infectious Diseases

Chickenpox   Mumps
Fifth Disease   Roseola
German Measles   Scarlet Fever
Hepatitis   Whooping Cough
Infectious Mononucleosis   "My Child Has Been Exposed
Lyme Disease   to . . ."
Measles

When the telephone conversation with a parent strongly suggests
the diagnosis of an infectious disease, most of the outlined information about that illness should be provided at the time of the call:
The usual course of illness, degree of contagion, incubation period,
and basic treatment should all be offered as a single discussion. This
helps to confirm or challenge the presumed diagnosis and provides
a predictable course for the parents to follow.

General
Principles

Common
Symptoms

Emergencies
and Traumas

Minor
Infections

Infectious
Diseases

Parenting
Concerns

Infant
Care

Chickenpox (Varicella)

Screening Questions

Background
- Name, age, sex?
- Specific symptoms?
- Current medications and treatments?
- General condition of the child?
- Chronic medical conditions?

Description

Chickenpox is suggested by a rash that itches and is described as small blisters (vesicles) on a red base and that begins on the trunk and abdomen and later spreads to the arms, legs, and face. The patient may have fever that is commonly low-grade. The lesions later develop into whitehead pimples (pustules) and eventually into scabs (blood crusts). Other symptoms are related to location of the lesions, *e.g.,* sore throat is common when lesions develop on the pharynx.

Contagion

- Children are considered contagious for 1 to 2 days prior to onset of rash and for approximately 5 days afterward. They are believed to be most contagious during the few days before the rash appears. Infected patients should avoid contact with others who have no past history of infection and who have not been immunized against this disease.
- Chickenpox is spread by virus from skin lesions and respiratory secretions.
- Individuals who are immunosuppressed because of chemotherapy, receipt of corticosteroids, or infection with human immunodeficiency virus (HIV) are at special risk for developing serious complications.

Jeffrey L. Brown: *Pediatric Telephone Medicine: Principles, Triage, and Advice,* Second Edition. Copyright © 1994 J. B. Lippincott Company

- Pregnant women with no previous history of disease or vaccination should be advised when contact with infected persons has occurred.

Incubation Period

- 10 to 21 days, but 14 days is usual.

Initial Treatment

- Antihistamines for itching and sedation.
- Acetaminophen for symptomatic relief of fever or pain. *Aspirin should be not be given.*
- Throat lozenges if sore throat is present in older children.
- Compresses or tepid bath for weeping lesions.
- Isolation for 5 to 7 days after lesions appear.
- Administration of oral acyclovir within 24 hours of onset of rash may be recommended for some patients.

Treatment of Contacts

- None for healthy individuals.
- Give varicella-zoster immune globulin (VZIG) to immunocompromised and other high-risk individuals.

Examination for

- Confirmation of diagnosis.
- Intractable symptoms.
- Severe systemic symptoms, especially when the child is described as looking toxic.
- Suggestion of secondary bacterial infection, especially impetigo.
- Vomiting or neurological symptoms during or after the acute illness.
- Eye lesions over the area of the pupil.

Parent Call-back Is Needed for

- Persistent, changing, worsening, anxiety-provoking, or specific symptoms as outlined above.

See Related Sections

The toxic child (p. 61), rash (p. 123), fever (p. 53), Reye's syndrome (p. 113).

Discussion

The use of oral antihistamines and topical agents, such as calamine lotion, for the *symptomatic relief* of discomfort associated with varicella lesions is less than optimal. Topical application of antihistamines should be avoided: Toxicity with development of neurological symptoms may result. Antihistamines are useful as a sedative, but relief from itching may be minimal. Some youngsters seem to gain more benefit from oral analgesics such as acetaminophen since itching may be the result of low-grade pain (similar to sunburn) rather than from histamine effect.

Impetigo is the most common complication and should be suspected when individual lesions become larger than the size of a dime. When the child complains of *severe burning pain* at the site of some lesions, consider the possibility of early secondary staphylococcal infection. Pain may occur 24 hours before lesions assume a typical impetigenous or bullous appearance.

Aspirin and other salicylates should never be given to children with chickenpox because of their known association with Reye's syndrome. This condition is suggested by neurological symptoms (headache, incoordination, slurred speech) and vomiting developing shortly after the acute infection has subsided.

Administration of corticosteroids, whether systemic, inhaled, or topical, may place the patient at risk for more severe illness. Varicella-zoster immune globulin (VZIG), acyclovir, or both may be recommended for use as soon as infection becomes apparent.

Conjunctival lesions usually disappear without treatment, but special attention should be paid to those that develop over the pupil. Ophthalmological consultation should be obtained to decrease the chances of corneal scarring.

Herpes zoster (shingles) occurs from reactivation of chickenpox virus from a previous infection. Chickenpox-like skin lesions develop in the band-like distribution of a sensory nerve. Herpes zoster is most commonly seen in adults but can also affect some children. Symptoms may persist for weeks. Infected individuals are believed to be contagious for about 1 week after the time of onset.

General Principles

Common Symptoms

Emergencies and Traumas

Minor Infections

Infectious Diseases

Parenting Concerns

Infant Care

General
Principles

Common
Symptoms

Emergencies
and Traumas

Minor
Infections

Infectious
Diseases

Parenting
Concerns

Infant
Care

Fifth Disease (Erythema Infectiosum, Parvovirus B19 Infection)

Screening Questions

Background
- Name, age, sex?
- Specific symptoms?
- Current medications and treatments?
- General condition of the child?
- Chronic medical conditions?

Description

Fifth disease is suggested by the appearance of a nonitching, bright red, slightly raised rash on the cheeks (slapped-cheek appearance) and a generalized rash consisting of flat or slightly raised lesions on the trunk; these may assume a lacy (morbilliform) pattern. Both rashes have a tendency to fade and recur (effervesce) over a period of hours. This rash is not usually associated with fever or other symptoms, and there is often no history of antecedent illness. Occasionally a low-grade fever or mild systemic complaints may be present. The eruption usually persists for 10 days but may last for as long as 5 weeks.

Contagion

- This viral illness is very contagious.
- Viral particles may be present in respiratory secretions or in blood.
- Children with fifth disease are *not* usually isolated because the course may be prolonged, symptoms are minimal, and the virus is thought to be most contagious before the rash appears.

Incubation Period

5 to 14 days (occasionally 21 days).

Jeffrey L. Brown: *Pediatric Telephone Medicine: Principles, Triage, and Advice,* Second Edition. Copyright © 1994 J. B. Lippincott Company

General
Principles

Common
Symptoms

Emergencies
and Traumas

Minor
Infections

Infectious
Diseases

Parenting
Concerns

Infant
Care

Initial Treatment

None.

Treatment of Contacts

- None.
- Pregnant women should be advised that this virus has been associated with fetal hydrops and fetal death. Overall risk for an exposed pregnant patient is believed to be small.
- Immunocompromised patients should be advised that this virus may cause an aplastic crisis.
- Exposed adults should be advised that this virus may cause arthritis.

Examination for

- Confirmation of diagnosis.

See Related Section

Rash (p. 123).

Discussion

This illness rarely causes significant morbidity for the infected child. Occasionally mild systemic symptoms or itching are present. More than 50 percent of adults show serologic evidence of previous parvovirus infection and have protective antibodies against the disease.

German Measles (Rubella)

Screening Questions

Background
- Name, age, sex?
- Specific symptoms?
- Current medications and treatments?
- General condition of the child?
- Chronic medical conditions?

Description

German measles is suggested by a red, irregular rash of individual, flat, or slightly raised lesions that begin on the face and later spread to cover the entire body. Children are not usually ill before the onset of the rash and usually have no associated respiratory symptoms. The temperature is low-grade (less than 101°F [38.4°C]). Many children have tender chains of lymph nodes in the back portion of the neck. The eruption generally fades by the third day and does not usually itch.

Contagion

- Children are contagious for approximately 7 days before and 5 days after appearance of the rash.
- Rubella is spread primarily in respiratory secretions, but the virus is also found in urine and stool.

Incubation Period

12 to 21 days (average 15 days).

General
Principles

Common
Symptoms

Emergencies
and Traumas

Minor
Infections

Infectious
Diseases

Parenting
Concerns

Infant
Care

Initial Treatment

- None is usually necessary.
- Acetaminophen for symptomatic relief of fever.
- The patient should avoid contact with pregnant women.

Treatment of Contacts

- *Pregnant women* who have been exposed to an infected child should have rubella titers drawn at the time of exposure to be repeated 2 weeks later. Some mothers may remain asymptomatic during active infection, especially if they have only partial protection from vaccination. Consider giving immune serum globulin when abortion would not be considered.
- Nonpregnant contacts require no treatment or evaluation.

Examination for

- Confirmation of diagnosis.

Parent Call-back Is Needed for

- Persistent, changing, worsening, anxiety-provoking, or specific symptoms.

See Related Section

Rash (p. 123).

Discussion

When a specific diagnosis of rubella is important, the clinician should never rely on physical examination alone. A rubella-like illness can be produced by many other viruses, and serologic diagnosis is necessary to confirm active infection or a past history of infection with subsequent immunity.

General
Principles

Common
Symptoms

Emergencies
and Traumas

Minor
Infections

Infectious
Diseases

Parenting
Concerns

Infant
Care

Hepatitis

Screening Questions

Background
- Name, age, sex?
- Specific symptoms?
- Current medications and treatments?
- General condition of the child?
- Chronic medical conditions?

Description

Hepatitis is an inflammation of the liver caused by different viral or toxic agents. Infection may cause jaundice, abdominal discomfort, and nonspecific symptoms such as fever, loss of appetite, and lethargy. When liver swelling is severe enough to cause destruction to the outflow of bile, dark-colored urine and light-colored stools may result. In mild cases, no signs or symptoms may be present. Diagnosis is made by obtaining a laboratory profile of liver function and viral antigens and antibodies.

Contagion

- The patient should initially be considered contagious while symptomatic until further laboratory tests can be obtained.

Incubation Period

- Variable, but usually at least 3 weeks.
- Serum hepatitis (type B) may have an incubation period as long as 6 months.

General
Principles

Common
Symptoms

Emergencies
and Traumas

Minor
Infections

Infectious
Diseases

Parenting
Concerns

Infant
Care

Initial Treatment

- Symptomatic.

Treatment of Contacts

- *Household and intimate contacts,* if not previously immunized, should receive gamma globulin or hepatitis B immune globulin when the diagnosis is confirmed to be infectious or serum hepatitis.
- *Casual or schoolroom contacts* require no treatment.

Examination for

- Confirmation of symptoms.
- Increasing signs of illness.

Parent Call-back Is Needed for

- Persistent, changing, worsening, anxiety-provoking, or specific symptoms as outlined above.

Discussion

Recent evidence suggests that both infectious and serum hepatitis viruses can be transmitted by the oral–fecal route (more common for infectious or type A hepatitis) and in body secretions (more common in serum or type B hepatitis). Strict hand washing after using the toilet and prior to eating are mandatory within the household, and common eating utensils should be avoided. Specific serologic testing may help to clarify the diagnosis, period of contagion, and treatment for these patients. Practical considerations suggest that all household and intimate contacts should be treated with gamma globulin or hepatitis B immune globulin (HBIG) unless they demonstrate evidence of immunity.

Infectious Mononucleosis (Epstein-Barr Virus Infection)

Screening Questions

Background
- Name, age, sex?
- Specific symptoms?
- Current medications and treatments?
- General condition of the child?
- Chronic medical conditions?

Description

Infectious mononucleosis is suggested by an upper respiratory tract infection, sore throat, enlarged lymph glands, and often an enlarged liver or spleen. Symptoms may be nonspecific and include fever, loss of appetite, and lethargy. Occasionally, jaundice or a measles-like rash may also be present.

The course of the illness is usually milder in younger children and may be no worse than a simple cold. Older children and adolescents may have an acute illness of approximately 7 days, but symptoms may last for a period of weeks.

Contagion

- The Epstein-Barr virus is spread in upper respiratory secretions.
- The patient is presumed to be most contagious while upper respiratory symptoms are present.
- Virus may be excreted for months after an acute infection.

Incubation Period

- 1 to 2 months.

General
Principles

Common
Symptoms

Emergencies
and Traumas

Minor
Infections

Infectious
Diseases

Parenting
Concerns

Infant
Care

Initial Treatment

- Acetaminophen for symptomatic relief of fever.
- Throat lozenges for throat pain.
- Avoidance of activities that can cause trauma to the abdomen.
- Patients with marked lymphoid swelling in the upper airway may benefit from a course of systemic steroids.

Treatment of Contacts

- None.

Examination for

- Confirmation of diagnosis.
- Persistence of symptoms.
- Obstructive breathing pattern.
- Toxic appearance.

Parent Call-back Is Needed for

- Persistent, changing, worsening, anxiety-provoking, or specific symptoms as outlined above.

See Related Sections

The toxic child (p. 61), fever (p. 53), pharyngitis (p. 77), upper respiratory infection (p. 81), rash (p. 123).

Discussion

Most parents associate this diagnosis with the prolonged illness commonly seen in teenagers and young adults. They are not aware that infection with the Epstein-Barr virus is common in nursery schools and day-care centers and that younger children usually have symptoms consistent with a simple cold. Most teenagers already have immunity to infection without a past history of previous disease. There has been concern in recent years that Epstein-Barr virus may cause chronic symptoms or reinfection in some individuals.

Active teenagers who develop infectious mononucleosis should avoid contact sports or other activities that place them at risk for sustaining abdominal trauma. An *enlarged spleen* (even if not palpable on examination) may persist for 6 weeks and might be more susceptible to rupture following a blow to the abdomen. Other activities should be limited only to the level of the child's tolerance.

General Principles

Common Symptoms

Emergencies and Traumas

Minor Infections

Infectious Diseases

Parenting Concerns

Infant Care

Lyme Disease

Screening Questions

Background
- Name, age, sex?
- Specific symptoms?
- Current medications and treatments?
- General condition of the child?
- Chronic medical conditions?

Description

Following the bite of a deer tick, a child may develop a spreading slightly raised red rash with a clearing center, known as erythema chronicum migrans (ECM). The rash may form either at the site of the bite or on another part of the body. Systemic symptoms of headache, muscle aches, fever, and joint pain may come and go over the next few weeks when patients are untreated. Weeks to months later, additional symptoms of arthritis (especially in large joints), facial weakness (Bell's palsy), meningitis, or other neurological signs may develop.

Contagion

None.

Incubation Period

Variable. From days to months following a tick bite.

Initial Treatment

- Antibiotics should be administered as soon as the diagnosis is believed to be likely.

Jeffrey L. Brown: *Pediatric Telephone Medicine: Principles, Triage, and Advice,* Second Edition. Copyright © 1994 J. B. Lippincott Company

217

General Principles

Common Symptoms

Emergencies and Traumas

Minor Infections

Infectious Diseases

Parenting Concerns

Infant Care

- Some physicians recommend treating all patients in areas endemic to Lyme disease with antibiotics as soon as a tick bite is noticed. Others treat only for suspected or confirmed disease.

Treatment of Contacts

None needed. This illness is not transmitted from one individual to another.

Evaluation Needed for

- Confirmation of diagnosis.
- Any rash suggestive of ECM.
- Signs or symptoms of arthritis.
- Neurological signs or symptoms.

Parent Call-back Is Needed for

- Persistent, changing, worsening, anxiety-provoking, or specific symptoms as outlined above.

Discussion

A history of tick bite may only be present in one-third of patients who develop Lyme disease. The offending tick is about the size of a sesame seed and can easily be missed on examination. *Treatment of tick bites* that occur in endemic areas is controversial. The risk for infection is believed to approximate 1 case per 100 bites. Ticks left in place for less than 24 hours before removal appear to create the least risk. *Prevention* of tick bites by dressing children in long sleeves and pants when practical, using repellents, and performing daily "tick checks" at bath time are the best methods. Diagnostic serologic tests can produce confusing results, and clinicians frequently treat on the basis of a presumptive diagnosis.

Untreated illness may mimic other bacterial, viral, collagen, and neurological conditions. Symptoms must be evaluated individually and as a group. Diagnosis is easily missed unless a *high index of suspicion* is maintained. *Treatment* of Lyme disease in the early stages with oral antibiotics is usually successful. In later stages parenteral medication may be required.

Measles (Rubeola)

Screening Questions

Background
- Name, age, sex?
- Specific symptoms?
- Current medications and treatments?
- General condition of the child?
- Chronic medical conditions?

Description

Measles is suggested by a generalized red rash that usually does not itch. It may be described as blotchy, irregular, and flat or slightly raised. It begins on the face and later spreads to the chest, abdomen, and extremities. It usually follows 3 to 5 days of upper respiratory tract infection, cough, conjunctivitis, and fever in the range of 101°F to 104°F (38.4°C to 40.0°C). The rash usually persists 4 to 7 days.

Contagion

- The greatest period of contagion occurs prior to the appearance of rash.
- The virus is usually spread by sneezing and coughing but may also be present in urine.
- Children should be isolated for at least 4 days after appearance of rash.

Incubation Period

Onset of symptoms usually begins 10 to 12 days after exposure.

Jeffrey L. Brown: *Pediatric Telephone Medicine: Principles, Triage, and Advice,* Second Edition. Copyright © 1994 J. B. Lippincott Company

General
Principles

Common
Symptoms

Emergencies
and Traumas

Minor
Infections

Infectious
Diseases

Parenting
Concerns

Infant
Care

Initial Treatment

- Acetaminophen for symptomatic relief of fever.
- Decongestants for symptomatic relief of upper respiratory tract infection.
- Dark glasses if the patient complains that light hurts the eyes.

Treatment of Contacts

- Give immune serum globulin when there is no past history of measles vaccination or measles illness.
- Unvaccinated children should be immunized with vaccine 8 weeks later.
- Previously vaccinated children require no treatment.

Examination for

- Confirmation of diagnosis.
- Evaluation of symptoms suggesting secondary infection.

Parent Call-back Is Needed for

- Persistent, changing, worsening, anxiety-provoking, or specific symptoms as outlined above.

See Related Sections

The toxic child (p. 61), fever (p. 53), upper respiratory infection (p. 81), lower respiratory infection (p. 67), otitis (p. 73), rash (p. 123).

Discussion

Complications of measles requiring antibiotics are common. These include otitis media and pneumonia. Viral encephalitis occurs in approximately 1 in 1000 patients and should be considered if signs and symptoms are compatible with this diagnosis.

Previously vaccinated patients with only partial immunity may develop *atypical measles syndromes*. The rash may be present with minimal symptoms, and fever may develop without rash. Individuals immunized

220

with older forms of vaccine, especially when administered with gamma globulin, may develop an eruption that suggests a rickettsial or allergic appearance. Those children immunized prior to their first birthday with older forms of vaccine or who received gamma globulin with earlier vaccines should be reimmunized using current schedules.

General
Principles

Common
Symptoms

Emergencies
and Traumas

Minor
Infections

Infectious
Diseases

Parenting
Concerns

Infant
Care

Mumps (Epidemic Parotitis)

Screening Questions

Background
- Name, age, sex?
- Specific symptoms?
- Current medications and treatments?
- General condition of the child?
- Chronic medical conditions?

Description

Mumps is characterized by tender swelling of the salivary glands. This gives the appearance of an ill-defined mass in front of one or both ears and persists for about 7 to 10 days. Ear pain made worse by chewing or swallowing is often present prior to or during the time of the swelling. The patient's temperature is variable; fever may be absent or as high as 104°F (40.0°C). Upper respiratory symptoms are frequently present. One-third of infected patients do not develop swelling of the salivary glands.

Contagion

- The child is considered contagious for 7 days prior to the onset of the first swelling and remains contagious until salivary gland swelling has disappeared, usually after about 1 week.
- The mumps virus is spread primarily by contact with respiratory secretions and saliva.

Incubation Period

- 12 to 24 days; 16 days average.

General
Principles

Common
Symptoms

Emergencies
and Traumas

Minor
Infections

**Infectious
Diseases**

Parenting
Concerns

Infant
Care

Initial Treatment

- Analgesics and decongestants for symptomatic relief of pain, fever, or runny nose.
- Isolation from others who have not had previous disease or vaccination.

Treatment of Contacts

- *Prepubertal children:* None.
- *Postpubertal males:* Immune serum globulin (gamma globulin) or mumps hyperimmune globulin may be useful.

Examination for

- Confirmation of diagnosis.
- Toxic appearance or neurological symptoms.
- Persistent abdominal pain.
- Testicular pain or swelling.

Parent Call-back Is Needed for

- Persistent, changing, worsening, anxiety-provoking, or specific symptoms as outlined above.

See Related Sections

The toxic child (p. 61), fever (p. 53), upper respiratory infection (p. 81).

Discussion

CLINICAL TIP. Mumps can be confused with tender swollen glands in the neck. Careful inspection will show that the facial swelling from mumps occurs in front of the ear; adenopathy occurs under the jaw line. A serum amylase level determination (usually elevated in mumps) may be used for a rapid, presumptive diagnosis.

Infectious parotitis is caused by the paramyxovirus. But other infectious organisms can cause similar symptoms. Conversely, patients can be infected with the mumps virus but never develop symptoms of salivary gland swelling.

Complications of mumps that require prompt evaluation include:

- *Encephalitis,* suggested by the sudden onset of vomiting, headache, stiff neck, and lethargy.
- *Pancreatitis,* suggested by sudden onset of mid- or upper abdominal pain, often with vomiting.
- *Orchitis,* suggested by testicular pain, especially in postpubertal youngsters.

General
Principles

Common
Symptoms

Emergencies
and Traumas

Minor
Infections

Infectious
Diseases

Parenting
Concerns

Infant
Care

Roseola (Exanthem Subitum, Sixth Disease)

Screening Questions

Background
- Name, age, sex?
- Specific symptoms?
- Current medications and treatments?
- Chronic medical conditions?

Description

Roseola is suggested when a young child has 2 to 3 days of high spiking fevers. A return to normal temperature is followed by the appearance of a nonitching red, flat, or slightly raised rash that covers the entire body; it may be most prominent over the trunk. The eruption lasts about 2 days and most commonly affects children under age 2 years. Symptoms of an upper respiratory tract infection, swelling of the lymph nodes in the back of the neck, irritability, and loss of appetite may be present. Other children may be virtually without symptoms. These young children may appear disproportionately well during episodes of fever even when temperatures range from 104°F to 106°F (40°C to 41°C).

Some children infected with the same causative agent, human herpes virus 6 (HHV-6), may develop high fever without rash, rash without fever, and asymptomatic infection. Febrile convulsions are a not uncommon complication of infection.

Contagion

- Incubation period is believed to be 5 to 15 days.
- The period of contagion is believed to be greatest during the time of fever before the rash occurs. However, it is unusual to identify the source of infection for an affected child.
- Affected children are not usually isolated unless the diagnosis is in doubt.

General
Principles

Common
Symptoms

Emergencies
and Traumas

Minor
Infections

Infectious
Diseases

Parenting
Concerns

Infant
Care

Initial Treatment

Acetaminophen for symptomatic relief of fever.

Treatment of Contacts

None.

Examination for

- Confirmation of diagnosis.
- Toxic or ill appearance.
- Febrile convulsions.

Parent Call-back Is Needed for

- Persistent, changing, worsening, anxiety-provoking, or specific symptoms as outlined above.

See Related Sections

Fever (p. 53), rash (p. 123), convulsion (pp. 57, 163).

Discussion

The rash of roseola can easily be confused with those of *other viral exanthems* and is usually diagnosed by clinical history alone. If the child was placed on antibiotics during the febrile period for otitis media or another presumed bacterial infection, it may be difficult to differentiate this rash from a *drug eruption*. When the rash is described as itchy or hive-like, the antibiotic should be discontinued or changed and antihistamines administered.

Morbidity results from the anxiety of uncertain diagnosis when there is no obvious source for infection. HHV-6 infection has been shown to be responsible for febrile convulsions in young children even when the typical exanthem does not appear.

General
Principles

Common
Symptoms

Emergencies
and Traumas

Minor
Infections

Infectious
Diseases

Parenting
Concerns

Infant
Care

Scarlet Fever (Scarlatina)

Screening Questions

Background
- Name, age, sex?
- Specific symptoms?
- Current medications and treatments?
- General condition of the child?
- Chronic medical conditions?

Description

Scarlet fever is suggested by a diffuse coarse redness of the skin that fades on pressure and is most prominent in the arm creases and in the groin. It is sometimes described as looking similar to a sunburn. The tongue may be red or coated. The rash usually occurs shortly after the child has developed fever, sore throat, and swollen glands. Vomiting is frequently present on the first day.

This illness is caused by the Group A beta-hemolytic streptococcus. Complications can include otitis media, infection of the lymph nodes (adenitis), sepsis, rheumatic fever, and kidney involvement (acute glomerulonephritis). As the rash gradually disappears, patients may develop peeling skin, especially on the palms and soles.

Contagion

- This illness is spread in respiratory secretions.
- Children should be isolated until the diagnosis is confirmed and until they have been treated with antibiotics for at least 24 hours.

Incubation Period

Onset of symptoms usually occurs within 3 days of exposure.

Jeffrey L. Brown: *Pediatric Telephone Medicine: Principles, Triage, and Advice,*
Second Edition. Copyright © 1994 J. B. Lippincott Company

General
Principles

Common
Symptoms

Emergencies
and Traumas

Minor
Infections

Infectious
Diseases

Parenting
Concerns

Infant
Care

Initial Treatment

- Acetaminophen for symptomatic relief of fever.
- Throat lozenges for sore throat.
- Antibiotics after the patient has been examined.

Treatment of Contacts

Symptomatic contacts should have throat cultures taken. Antibiotics may be started before culture results are available.

Examination for

- Rash suggestive of scarletina with or without other symptoms.

Parent Call-back Is Needed for

- Persistent, changing, worsening, anxiety-provoking, or specific symptoms as outlined above.

See Related Sections

The toxic child (p. 61), upper respiratory infection (p. 81), pharyngitis (p. 77), fever (p. 53), rash (p. 123).

Discussion

Some children develop a mild variant of this illness with a typical scarlet-fever-like rash and positive throat culture but few other symptoms. Affected children may return to school when they feel well and have been taking antibiotics for at least 24 hours. Persistence of rash is not an indication for isolation.

General
Principles

Common
Symptoms

Emergencies
and Traumas

Minor
Infections

Infectious
Diseases

Parenting
Concerns

Infant
Care

Whooping Cough (Pertussis)

Screening Questions

Background
- Name, age, sex?
- Specific symptoms?
- Current medications and treatments?
- General condition of the child?
- Chronic medical conditions?

Description

Whooping cough is a bacterial infection of both the upper and lower airways that has the initial appearance of the common cold. The child later develops a severe, persistent, and unusual cough that occurs in short bursts throughout the day. The coughing fit cannot be controlled and may cause vomiting. Small children may become dusky during these episodes. When the child takes a deep breath at the end of the coughing fit, a breathing-in "whoop" may be heard. High fever is not common. Severely ill children may have breath-holding and convulsions. Immunized individuals may develop a mild and atypical version of this disease.

Contagion

- This illness is most contagious before the onset of cough when only runny nose is present.
- The child should be considered contagious during the time that she is coughing.

Incubation

- 7 to 10 days from the time of exposure.

Jeffrey L. Brown: *Pediatric Telephone Medicine: Principles, Triage, and Advice,*
Second Edition. Copyright © 1994 J. B. Lippincott Company

231

General
Principles

Common
Symptoms

Emergencies
and Traumas

Minor
Infections

Infectious
Diseases

Parenting
Concerns

Infant
Care

Initial Treatment

- Decongestants and antipyretics for symptomatic relief.
- Antibiotics if the diagnosis is presumed.

Treatment of Contacts

- *Household and intimate contacts* should be treated with prophylactic antibiotics.
- *Children less than 7 years old* may require a booster diptheria,
  pertussis, tetanus (DPT) immunization.
- *All contacts* should report respiratory symptoms that develop
  within 2 weeks of exposure.

Examination for

- Confirmation of diagnosis.
- Worsening respiratory symptoms.
- Toxic appearance.

Parent Call-back Is Needed for

- Persistent, changing, worsening, anxiety-provoking, or specific
  symptoms as outlined above.

See Related Sections

The toxic child (p. 61), fever (p. 53), upper respiratory infection (p. 81),
cough (p. 65).

Discussion

Unfortunately, whooping cough has become more prevalent during the
past few years. Controversy about the potential dangers of pertussis vaccine has encouraged some parents to refuse consent for immunization.

Individuals who were previously immunized may develop only mild
illness. Adults with pertussis may commonly be misdiagnosed as having
chronic bronchitis. When the infected individual is of baby-sitting age,
this may prove dangerous to unimmunized or partially immunized infants
who are at greatest risk for the most serious complications.

General
Principles

Common
Symptoms

Emergencies
and Traumas

Minor
Infections

Infectious
Diseases

Parenting
Concerns

Infant
Care

"My Child Has Been Exposed to . . ."

Screening Questions

Background
- Name, age, sex?
- Specific symptoms?
- Current medications and treatments?
- General condition of the child?
- Chronic medical conditions?

Acquired Immunodeficiency Syndrome (AIDS)

No treatment is available or necessary. Although the infecting human immunodeficiency virus (HIV) may be present in any body fluid, transmission is extremely uncommon except by sexual contact, sharing a needle, or receiving blood products from an infected individual. Nonsexual household contacts of infected individuals do not appear to have a greater risk of developing this illness. Casual contact with an AIDS patient should not be cause for concern.

Chickenpox (Varicella)

No treatment is usually necessary. If the exposed child has not been immunized and has severe underlying illness, is immunocompromised, or is receiving corticosteroids, prophylactic administration of zoster immune globulin should be considered and acyclovir given at the first sign of rash.

German Measles (Rubella)

No treatment is necessary. Symptoms are usually mild in unimmunized patients. Immunized patients will probably not contract the disease.

Jeffrey L. Brown: *Pediatric Telephone Medicine: Principles, Triage, and Advice*, Second Edition. Copyright © 1994 J. B. Lippincott Company

233

Head Lice (Pediculosis Capitus)

The exposed child should be examined at 1-week intervals for the presence of eggs. No treatment should be given unless infection occurs.

Hepatitis

Unimmunized exposed children should receive gamma globulin or hepatitis B immune globulin if the infected contact lives in the same house or is an intimate friend. No treatment is necessary for school or casual contacts.

Impetigo

No treatment is necessary unless the exposed child develops a rash that has the appearance of blisters (vessicles), pimples (pustules), or scabs (blood crusts).

Infectious Mononucleosis

No treatment is available or necessary.

Lyme Disease

No treatment is necessary. This infection is not transmitted person-to-person.

Measles (Rubeola)

No treatment is necessary if the patient has been immunized or previously had the disease. Immune serum globulin is recommended if the child has no immunological protection.

Meningitis

Many different microorganisms can cause meningitis. The parent of the exposed youngster should attempt to learn the causative agent before seeking advice. If the contact had viral meningitis, no treatment is necessary. If the illness was caused by *Haemophilus influenzae B* or meningococcus, prophylactic antibiotics should be prescribed for unimmunized children.

Mumps (Infectious Parotitis)

Treatment is necessary if the child has not previously had the disease or is unimmunized. Immune serum globulin may be recommended for susceptible postpubertal males.

Pinworm

If contact has been casual, asymptomatic children should receive no treatment. Household and intimate contacts should be treated at the same time as the infected patient.

Pneumonia

Many infectious agents can cause pneumonia, but they will not always cause the same symptoms in each person. An upper respiratory tract infection, sore throat, or earache may result after exposure to a patient ill with pneumonia. No prophylactic treatment is indicated.

Ringworm

This skin infection has a low degree of contagion. No treatment is necessary.

Scarlet Fever (Scarletina)

Treatment is the same as for strep throat. (See discussion below.)

Streptococcal Sore Throat (Strep Throat)

Symptomatic exposed children should have a throat culture taken and be treated if the culture is positive. Antibiotics may be started while culture results are pending.

General Principles

Common Symptoms

Emergencies and Traumas

Minor Infections

Infectious Diseases

Parenting Concerns

Infant Care

Whooping Cough (Pertussis)

If contact has been intimate, even previously immunized children should be started on prophylactic antibiotics.

Notes

General
Principles

Common
Symptoms

Emergencies
and Traumas

Minor
Infections

Infectious
Diseases

Parenting
Concerns

Infant
Care

General
Principles

Common
Symptoms

Emergencies
and Traumas

Minor
Infections

Infectious
Diseases

Parenting
Concerns

Infant
Care

Notes

Notes

Notes

Section VI

Common Parenting Concerns

Common Complaints Received
  by Age Group
Basic Principles when
  Discussing Behavior with
  Parents

Abbreviated Discussions of
  Common Pediatric Problems

Many of the concerns discussed in this chapter are more appropriately discussed with parents at the time of a child's routine physical examination. It is not uncommon, however, for parents to call asking for advice when anxiety precludes waiting until the next scheduled visit. A sampling of relatively brief responses to these common concerns has been included for reference.

Minor
Infections

Infectious
Diseases

Parenting
Concerns

Infant
Care

Common Complaints Received by Age Group

1 Month

Colicky pain. See infant colic (p. 101).
  Others. See infant care (p. 261).

3 Months

Teething. Although the first two teeth do not usually erupt until age 6 to 8 months, infants may show signs of early teething at about 10 weeks. These babies are described as drooling and biting their fists. A morning cough may result from secretions accumulating at the back of the throat, especially when the infant is in the supine position. These symptoms may be mistaken for an upper respiratory tract infection. No treatment is necessary.

6 Months

Crying episodes. Fretfulness, crying, and awakening during the night may be caused by *true teething.* Topical anesthetics may provide relief for brief periods; acetaminophen is more useful because it is effective for 3 to 4 hours. Rubbing the infant's gums without medication is also soothing.

7 Months

The baby is "spoiled." Coincidental with becoming motile (crawling and pulling to standing) the infant may come to regard a playpen or crib as a cage and vigorously protest a parent leaving the room. This may be misinterpreted as "spoiled" behavior but probably reflects frustration at not being able to exercise a newly learned skill. No corrective action is necessary.

General
Principles

Common
Symptoms

Emergencies
and Traumas

Minor
Infections

Infectious
Diseases

Parenting
Concerns

Infant
Care

12 to 15 Months

Poor eating. The normal eating pattern for toddlers is to eat one main meal a day, together with small multiple feedings. (See poor eating p. 252.)

Poor sleeping. See sleeping problems (p. 253).

Temper tantrums. Children should be given little attention while they are having temper tantrums, so as to not reinforce this behavior. When the tantrum has ended, they should be treated in a loving way (without giving in to the desire that precipitated the behavior). The child is then being rewarded for stopping. Temper tantrums may become less frequent when children become better at verbalizing their thoughts (at about $2\frac{1}{2}$ years old).

$2\frac{1}{2}$ to $3\frac{1}{2}$ Years

Variable behavior with compulsive traits. Periods of compliant behavior alternating with cranky, irritable, and demanding behavior are normal.

Bedtime and eating rituals often occur together with temper outbursts when the child's expectations are not met.

Ritualistic or compulsive behavior may reflect the child's attempt to control his environment because his borderline skills have caused a feeling of insecurity. Intervention is necessary only when this behavior is intentionally manipulative.

Common potential stresses may be blamed for normal behavior variations. These include starting nursery school, the birth of a sibling, family relocation, sick grandparents, and parents who are beginning or changing jobs.

A child's *mood swings* may coincide with those of his parents. These may reinforce one another. Having an awareness of the problem is helpful.

Make the child's day as *predictable* as possible: Some children who do poorly in a three-times-a-week nursery school will improve behavior when attending every day.

Avoid confrontations when possible, but consistently be firm about more important matters.

$3\frac{1}{2}$ to $4\frac{1}{2}$ Years

Demandingly inquisitive.

Insist on performing tasks by themselves.

Accept this period as necessary for combined learning and assertiveness.

244

6 to 7 Years

Verbalization of anger directed at parents. Conformity required by first grade learning situations may provoke anger directed at parents when the child returns home from school. Awareness is necessary for parental understanding.

7 to 9 Years

Peer pressure causing conformity. Desire to conform to a group should be considered normal. Associated stress may cause unexplained mood swings.

School difficulties. Poor academic skills may cause behavior problems when children try to avoid tasks that are difficult for them. Contacting the child's teacher may be helpful.

10 to 12 Years

Apathetic and moody. Prepubertal youngsters are too old to comfortably participate at younger children's activities but are too young for adolescent activities. They may withdraw socially and appear to have a lack of interest. Parents should try to promote activities that reinforce strengths rather than try to make the child "well rounded."

Teenage Years

Exaggerated emotional responses. Hormones and environmental factors may cause teenagers to exaggerate their responses to verbal and physical stimuli. Also, previous experience does not create a buffer for daily events. Their world is either awful or terrific. Parents should try to keep them on an even keel by responding in a "mature" adult way.

Erratic and confrontational behavior. Adolescent behavior has many similarities to that of toddlers: Teens are learning how to socialize, feel comfortable with their minds and bodies, and experiment with boundaries. Parents must use a skillful combination of consistency, love, reassurance, and discipline.

Most important, they should not mistake their child's grown-up appearance as a sign that he or she will think and act in a mature way. Parents also need a sense of humor.

General Principles

Common Symptoms

Emergencies and Traumas

Minor Infections

Infectious Diseases

Parenting Concerns

Infant Care

Basic Principles when Discussing Behavior with Parents

Screening Questions

- *Duration.* How long has the problem been present?
- *Activities affected.* Does the problem interfere with home life, social relationships, school work, or all of these?
- *Environmental problems.* Have there been any recent problems at home (financial or family-related strife)?
- *Parent's intuition.* If you had to pick one reason for the problem, what would you pick?

Conference Necessary for

- Extreme parental anxiety.
- Problems described as chronic or long-term.
- Problems that extend from one sphere (home, peers, and school) into another: Help for problems in one sphere is elective; help for problems in two spheres is strongly recommended; help for problems in three spheres is mandatory.

Discussion

Most behavior problems that worry parents reflect normal childhood development. Unrealistic parental expectations for the child must be corrected. When a parent describes the problem as chronic, or believes that it involves more than one sphere of the child's daily activities (family, work, and peers), the child's normal defense mechanisms may not be compensating for her stress, and a complete evaluation is necessary. Telephone advice should be given concerning the immediate crisis, and an appointment should be made to discuss the full scope of the problem.

Jeffrey L. Brown: *Pediatric Telephone Medicine: Principles, Triage, and Advice,* Second Edition. Copyright © 1994 J. B. Lippincott Company

General Principles

Common Symptoms

Emergencies and Traumas

Minor Infections

Infectious Diseases

Parenting Concerns

Infant Care

Basic Principles for Discussing Behavior-related Problems

- *Delineate the problem.* Choose the three or four most troublesome aspects of behavior and focus attention on them. This decreases parental anxiety by constructing boundaries to work within, rather than allowing parents to have the abstract feeling that "things aren't going well."
- *Establish precipitating factors.* When a behavior problem occurs following a major stress such as a parent losing a job, or the child changing schools, examine this stress factor first.
- *Question the child.* Children may be a good source of information concerning their own problems. Parents should question them in a nonthreatening, nonaccusatory way. A useful preface to questioning might be "I've been feeling badly for you; I can see that things haven't been going well. Is there anything you would like to talk with me about?"
- *Give parents time off.* Parenting young children is more strenuous mentally and physically than most other occupations. As with other jobs, parents need to look forward to having time off. When the relationship between a parent and a young child is going poorly, the parent may respond by feeling guilty and leave the child with a sitter less often. When the parent spends almost no time alone, time off should be arranged on a *regular schedule.*
- *Develop a punishment.* Establishing an effective and suitable punishment is important for maintaining discipline. The specific punishment depends on age and personality. Many believe that hitting should be avoided when possible but might be considered for actions that are repetitively dangerous or are openly defiant. A more useful punishment is to separate the child by placing him in his room or in a semi-isolated area with the admonition "I would prefer that you stay here with us, but when you behave this way, you will have to stay by yourself."
- *Be predictable.* Discipline should be predictable so that the child can avoid it with proper behavior. Well-adjusted children are found in both liberal and strict households when extremes are avoided, parents are not hypocritical, and their responses to the child's behavior are consistent.
- *Reward normal behavior.* Children frequently receive more attention for acting out than when they behave normally. They may be yelled at and punished for throwing food at the table but receive

248

only a silent sigh of relief when they eat quietly. Children should be punished with as little emotion as possible but receive lots of encouragement and praise for good behavior. Extra attention should be given for activities that are considered "normal" to reinforce this behavior.

General
Principles

Common
Symptoms

Emergencies
and Traumas

Minor
Infections

Infectious
Diseases

Parenting
Concerns

Infant
Care

General
Principles

Common
Symptoms

Emergencies
and Traumas

Minor
Infections

Infectious
Diseases

Parenting
Concerns

Infant
Care

Abbreviated Discussions of Common Pediatric Problems

Toilet Training

Children are neurologically ready to be toilet-trained when they are able to run (age 18 to 20 months). However, not all children in this age group are psychologically ready. When children understand cause and effect well (about $2\frac{1}{2}$ years), they are more likely to toilet-train in a consistent way.

A potty-chair is preferred to a "trainer seat" that snaps onto an adult toilet seat. The child can gain access without parental help and it allows feet to touch the ground.

Parents should familiarize the child with the potty-chair when they are not hurried. Reading materials, "potty toys," or charts with stars may be used as incentives. Once the child will sit on the seat, either with or without a diaper, training may begin in earnest.

Every time the child soils a diaper, the parent should offer a gentle, unemotional directive. This should consist only of an acknowledgment of displeasure: "I don't want you to go in your diaper anymore. Now you're supposed to use the potty." If parents become overly emotional when the child soils a diaper, it is not long before this becomes a means of getting attention. Also, because children have many more incidents of diaper soiling than potty use, more attention is gained on a regular basis from stooling in the wrong place.

When the child does go to the bathroom in the proper place, much positive reinforcement should be used. This can consist of hugging, kissing, clapping, charts with stars, or other similar devices.

In summary, the child should use a potty instead of a trainer seat. The parent should negatively acknowledge a soiled diaper but offer lots of praise for the child's using the toilet. Setbacks should be expected and no time limit should be set for training.

Bed Wetting (Enuresis)

Bed wetting should not be considered a significant problem unless the child is older than age 6 years. Approximately one in five youngsters at

General
Principles

Common
Symptoms

Emergencies
and Traumas

Minor
Infections

Infectious
Diseases

Parenting
Concerns

Infant
Care

age 6 continues to wet the bed. Enuretic children often have a family history of childhood enuresis.

Children with a history of frequent daytime wetting, or those who have never been dry at night, should be evaluated for the possibility of an underlying urologic abnormality. If they can remain dry during the daytime or have had periods when they have been dry all night, the chance of underlying organic illness is small.

Advice

- Restrict fluids after dinner. When children wish to drink just prior to bedtime, most will be content just taking sips.
- Children should be asked to urinate just prior to going to sleep. Parents may wish to bring the children to the bathroom in the late evening until they are trained.
- If these simple measures fail, a calendar may be used on which dry nights are starred. A reward may follow when boxes on the chart have been filled. Little acknowledgment should be given when the child wakes up wet, but dry mornings should be treated with much bravado and praise.
- *Medications* such as imipramine or DDAVP nasal spray might be considered for youngsters older than age 6 years when other measures have failed.
- *Training devices,* such as electric alarms, are effective, but some children find them degrading.
- *Imagery and self-hypnosis* are also effective and should be discussed as an option with selected families at in-person conferences.

Poor Eating

Parents first complain of poor eating when their child is between *12 and 15 months old.* At that time, most children change their eating habits to eat one substantial meal a day in addition to *small frequent feedings.* These should not be considered snacks, and *snack foods* should not be used. The time of the large meal varies from day to day, and it may be skipped entirely.

This change in eating pattern occurs because the rate of growth decreases at the end of the first year. During the first year, most children increase their weight by 300 percent. During the second year, weight increases by less than 25 percent; more weight may be gained during the first 3 months of life than during the entire second year.

This pattern may persist until the age of 6 years. When weight gain has been adequate, parents should not be concerned. Three meals a day should be offered, but the quantity of food consumed should be at the child's discretion. Foods offered throughout the day should consist of those that were rejected at meal times rather than traditional snack foods.

A common parental error when *choosing foods* is to assume that the child likes the same foods as the parents. Parents who never eat brussel sprouts may not bring them home because they don't consider them to be a real "food." However, their child who rejects "kiddy foods" like peas and corn may think brussel sprouts are terrific. It was once said that "if children picked the food, they might think that adults were picky eaters." Parents also forget that children eat smaller portions than they do.

Multivitamins may be prescribed, along with reassurance, if parents are advised that these preparations are not usually necessary and will not increase the child's appetite. Remind parents that if the child looks healthy, the chance of a significant nutritional problem is minimal.

Poor Sleeping

Many children believed to be poor sleepers have *normal sleeping patterns*. Until the age of $2\frac{1}{2}$ children commonly sleep a total of about 12 hours per day. The most usual pattern is to sleep from 8:00 P.M. to 6:00 A.M. or from 10:00 P.M. to 8:00 A.M. with 2 hours of nap time. Some few children will sleep 12 hours at night with no nap. Parents of children with these normal patterns may complain that their child awakens too early, falls asleep too late, or won't nap. They need only reassurance.

Sleeping aids such as pacifiers, bottles, and *physical aids* such as rocking and holding should be avoided during the time the child actually falls asleep. Most children awaken during the night, but those who use sleeping aids can't fall asleep again until they have help. When children become used to falling asleep without the parent present, there is a better chance that they can fall asleep again effortlessly.

Night bottles should be avoided. Bottles that contain milk or juice may cause caries. Also the child awakens more frequently because of a wet diaper and then can't return to sleep without receiving a new bottle.

A gradually *increased time of crying* alone should be allowed for children who are poor sleepers. Parents who are concerned about the psychological effects of three or four nights of "abandonment" should weigh them against the psychological effects that their own sleep deprivation will have on their next year of effective parenting.

Self-soothing mechanisms can only occur when children can get themselves back to sleep. The children should first fall asleep in an empty

General Principles

Common Symptoms

Emergencies and Traumas

Minor Infections

Infectious Diseases

Parenting Concerns

Infant Care

General
Principles

Common
Symptoms

Emergencies
and Traumas

Minor
Infections

Infectious
Diseases

Parenting
Concerns

Infant
Care

room with no one present, so that when they awaken during the night they do not require outside aids to fall back to sleep.

Circadian rhythms. Even small infants develop light–dark cycles. Nighttime sleeping should be done in a dark room; avoid of bright lights when the child is up during the night. Daytime naps should be taken in a brightly lit room.

Fearfulness

Two- and 3-year-olds may become afraid of darkness, shadows, and "monsters in the closet." These children have suddenly become aware that things in their environment may harm them, but they aren't sure which ones. This causes them to focus on abstract concerns. Simple re-assurance may be given by saying, "There are a lot of things that look scary, but you don't have to worry about this one." Avoid long conversa-tions that give the child undue attention for being scared.

Four- and 5-year-olds worry about intrusions into the house, especial-ly burglers and fires. Simple reassurance is all that is necessary.

Six- to 8-year-olds worry about bodily harm outside the house, espe-cially kidnappers. Reassurance given together with rules for proper safe-ty should be given.

Shyness

Parents may have the misconception that all children are outgoing and social. They may worry when their child does not actively participate with other children. At an adult social gathering, some stand off by them-selves, others aggressively introduce themselves, and most are a little shy but make conversation when approached. Children behave in a similar way. Those children who are shy to the point of not interacting socially at all may have a simple maturational problem or might fall into one of these normal categories. A complete history is necessary for proper eval-uation.

The Middle Child

The middle family child is told he is "too babyish" or "not old enough" when he tries to copy his younger and older siblings. Help him to find a place for himself by reinforcing those areas where he is strongest and con-centrating on them. This should be a more important objective than mak-ing him "well-rounded."

Sex Education

When parents request literature concerning sex-related matters, they should visit the local bookstore or library, survey available stock, and choose a book that they will feel comfortable reading with their youngster. An explicit, illustrated reference may be appropriate in one home but equally inappropriate in another. Similarly, an overly simplistic reference would be out of place in a home where frank discussions are commonplace.

Death of a Family Member or Friend

Advice given to parents about how to deal with their child after the death of a family member or friend depends on family structure, educational level, and age of the child. The following suggestions may be helpful.

Be truthful when discussing what happens after a person dies. Children may be told that "no one knows what happens after a person dies, but we believe that. . . ." If children are given an explanation that is not believed by the parents, they may sense the untruth and believe that death is so terrible that no one will tell them what really happens.

Allow children to be present during the *mourning ritual* if it is practical, appropraite for age and temperament, and thought to be in good taste. A good test would be to decide if the child would be allowed to attend a happy family function of almost equal importance, such as a wedding. Some children may feel less secure when separated from grieving family members. Keeping children with the family makes them feel part of the family structure and helps to keep the emotions of other family members in proper perspective.

Question children about their feelings and be empathetic with them. If they are angry or sad, explain that this is normal and to be expected.

Ambivalent Feelings of Working Mothers

Because of social attitudes and financial pressures, a large percentage of mothers with young children are actively employed. Many have ambivalent feelings because they want to assume a conventional mothering role but also feel a responsibility to pursue intellectual or career-oriented objectives. When the family's financial situation makes maternal employment necessary, or when part-time employment is feasible, the decision is somewhat easier. However, when the mother has true freedom of choice, she is best advised to choose the option that makes her feel the *least guilty,* rather than the one she prefers most. It may also be difficult

General
Principles

Common
Symptoms

Emergencies
and Traumas

Minor
Infections

Infectious
Diseases

Parenting
Concerns

Infant
Care

for mothers to separate their own feelings from those of their relatives and friends. The homemaker who spends most of her day wishing that she were doing something else may eventually come to resent her child and will usually be most happy if she returns to her employed job. The mother who spends much of her day worrying about her child's care while at her place of employment should most probably return home.

Notes

General
Principles

Common
Symptoms

Emergencies
and Traumas

Minor
Infections

Infectious
Diseases

Parenting
Concerns

Infant
Care

Notes

Notes

Notes

General Principles

Common Symptoms

Emergencies and Traumas

Minor Infections

Infectious Diseases

Parenting Concerns

Infant Care

260

Care of Newborn Infants

Each medical facility may wish to distribute instruction sheets on newborns to parents during prenatal conferences, at the hospital, or by mail when scheduling the first well-baby examination. These instruction sheets greatly reduce the number of questions asked by telephone during the baby's first few weeks of life. An example of typical advice that might be contained in patient handouts or offered to parents of newborn infants over the telephone is outlined in this section for reference. It should be modified to conform with an individual clinician's preferences. This information is also useful for staff when instructing patients over the telephone.

General
Principles

Common
Symptoms

Emergencies
and Traumas

Minor
Infections

Infectious
Diseases

Parenting
Concerns

Infant
Care

Infant Care

■ When To Call the Doctor

Parents should be instructed to call under the following circumstances.
- *Fever.* If the baby has a rectal temperature of 101°F (38.2°C) or higher (only rectal temperatures should be considered accurate).
- *Poor general appearance.* If the baby appears limp, has poor color, or is difficult to arouse.
- *Poor feeding.* If the baby refuses to suck or feed two or three times in a row.
- *Vomiting.* If the baby throws up most of its feedings.
- *Diarrhea.* If the baby has frequent watery bowel movements.
- *Jaundice.* If the baby looks very yellow, pumpkin-colored, or has yellow palms, soles, or abdomen.
- *Anxiety.* If the baby seems to be ill or if the parent feels frightened about the baby's symptoms or general appearance.
- *Calling instructions.* When calling for an emergency, the office receptionist or service operator should be told, "This is an emergency!" so that there will be no misunderstanding about the level of concern. If the call is not an emergency, parents should ask when the doctor or nurse is most likely to call back.

■ Breast Feeding

Breast feeding is the preferred method for feeding the baby. Comfortable nursing may not be easy at first, as both mother and baby adjust to each other. Most mothers and babies develop a reasonable feeding schedule within 2 weeks. Mothers should not be overly concerned even when the baby does not seem interested in nursing at first or there does not seem to be much milk during the first few days.

A nursing position comfortable to the mother should be recommended. The baby should directly face the breast, abdomen to abdomen. The

General
Principles

Common
Symptoms

Emergencies
and Traumas

Minor
Infections

Infectious
Diseases

Parenting
Concerns

Infant
Care

mother's hand used to present the breast to the baby should be placed suf-
ficiently back from the nipple so that the baby can latch on to as much of
the colored part of the nipple (the areola) as possible. Milk is actually
squeezed from the breast, and if only the tip of the nipple is offered, sore-
ness and poor feeding will result. The baby's mouth should be guided to
the breast by holding his or her head from behind. Avoid pushing on the
baby's cheek since the *rooting reflex* may cause the baby to turn toward
the pressure of the mother's hand rather than toward the breast. Before
removing the baby from the breast, the mother should gently break the
baby's suction by placing a finger in the corner of the baby's mouth. If the
baby has difficulty taking the breast because it is *engorged* (swollen), a
small amount of milk can be expressed by squeezing the areola between
two fingers before the baby begins nursing. This procedure can also be
used if the baby misses a feeding and engorged breasts feel uncomfortable. Many hand-operated, battery-operated, and electric breast pumps
are available to help *express milk.*

The *length of time* required for a baby to complete a feeding is variable. Babies get most of the milk during the first 10 minutes, and in most
cases a feeding will be completed within 20 minutes. But small, frequent
feedings may be necessary if nipples are sore, if only small amounts of
milk are being produced or if the baby is not nursing well. It may be helpful to alternate the starting breast at each feeding. A safety pin can be
placed on the bra strap of the starting side as a reminder.

Sore nipples can be treated with a bland ointment such as A & D or by
coating them with a small amount of expressed breast milk and allowing
them to air-dry. Leaving the flaps of the nursing bra open and wearing
loose-fitting cotton clothing is a practical solution. If one particular area
of the nipple is sore from the pressure of the baby's sucking, changing or
alternating nursing positions should be helpful.

If the baby *seems unsatisfied,* more frequent feedings (as often as
every 2 hours) should be tried. It is generally best to avoid giving a baby
sugar water or formula until breast feeding is well established (usually
by 2 weeks), although occasional bottles will not cause a problem in most
cases.

Breast-feeding mothers should eat a *healthy diet* and drink plenty of
fluids. If a mother's urine becomes dark and concentrated, insufficient
fluid intake should be suspected. All foods that create a balanced diet are
acceptable if eaten in moderation, but if the baby becomes irritable each
time a particular food is eaten, that food should be avoided for three or
four days and then reintroduced to see if symptoms disappear and then
reappear. *Medicines,* including laxatives, should be avoided unless a
physician or nurse has been contacted first. Rest and relaxation are important. Fatigue and worry are common causes of breast-feeding failure.

General
Principles

Common
Symptoms

Emergencies
and Traumas

Minor
Infections

Infectious
Diseases

Parenting
Concerns

Infant
Care

Many physicians recommend that parents give one dropperful per day of *baby vitamins* containing A, D, and C. If the baby does not drink any water, or if the water supply is not fluoridated, vitamins with *fluoride* may be prescribed. Nursing mothers should continue taking their prenatal vitamins.

■ Formula Feeding

When mothers cannot or choose not to breast feed their babies during the first year of life, *prepared infant formula with iron* should be used instead of cow's milk. At each feeding the baby will drink about half the number of ounces it weighs in pounds. For example, an 8-pound baby will usually drink about 4 ounces of formula (3 to 5 ounces) per feeding.

Ready-Nurser disposable bottled formula is the most expensive type, but it is very useful for emergencies, trips, and for supplemental feedings when nursing. These bottles may be kept at room temperature and offered to the baby without warming. Unused formula may be refrigerated after opening and offered at a second feeding.

If a *Ready-To-Feed* formula is used, the top of the can should be washed with soap and hot water and then poured immediately into a clean bottle. An opened can should be refrigerated and covered and can be used within 48 hours.

Concentrated and *powdered* formulas are less expensive. Powdered formula is especially convenient when making only a small amount of formula at a time, for example when supplementing breast feeding or traveling. Instructions on the label should be followed for proper dilution and mixing. Although *sterilization* is not always necessary, cleanliness in formula preparation is very important. Prepared bottles can be refrigerated or made one bottle at a time.

Most infants prefer formula that has been *warmed* to room temperature: Hot water from the faucet can be allowed to run over the bottle for a few minutes. Babies will not be harmed by drinking cold formula, and some (especially after age 6 months) prefer their bottles cold directly from the refrigerator. *Microwave warming* is *not* recommended. Not only can tightly sealed bottles explode, but scalding hot liquid may be inside a bottle that feels cool. If a bottle must be placed in the microwave, it should contain at least 4 ounces and have the top left open. Contents should be shaken thoroughly and the milk's temperature should be checked carefully before it is offered to the baby.

On hot days, *water* may occasionally be offered to the baby between regular feedings. *Sterilizing* for supplemental or formula use is not usu-

General
Principles

Common
Symptoms

Emergencies
and Traumas

Minor
Infections

Infectious
Diseases

Parenting
Concerns

Infant
Care

ally necessary, but when water quality is in doubt, boiling for 20 minutes during the first 3 months is recommended. *Lead* concentrations in tap water can be reduced by allowing early morning water to run freely before using and by loosely covering pots with a lid during heating. One teaspoon of *sugar* may be added to 4 ounces of water for taste.

Vitamins are contained in prepared infant formulas, and vitamin supplements are not necessary until formula is discontinued (usually at about age 1 year).

■ Feeding Schedules

There is no "right" feeding schedule that works best for all babies. A compromise between a strict feeding *schedule* and a *demand*-type feeding pattern is often effective. The baby can be fed every 2 to 4 hours during the daytime and allowed to sleep as long as he or she wishes at night. The baby's size and degree of fussiness can influence the frequency of feeding. At first, most babies feed once or twice each night. By age 3 months, about one-half of these infants sleep through the night (6 to 8 hours) without awakening.

■ Solid Foods

Breast milk or formula alone is the best diet for an infant during the first few months. Starting baby food early may cause allergies, changes in bowel movements, spitting up, or rashes. Early feedings may also cause the baby to gain too much weight too quickly. Adding solids to a baby's diet does not usually help them to sleep through the night sooner. If the baby seems hungry, he or she may be pacified by extra sucking, by drinking more milk or formula (either more frequently or in larger amounts), or by drinking plain water. Solids are not usually recommended until the baby is 4 to 6 months old, or until the baby weighs more than 15 pounds.

■ Bowel Movements

The baby's first stools contain *meconium,* a thick sticky substance that is tarry and dark brown in appearance. The *frequency* and *consistency* of the baby's later bowel movements may vary from day to day. Some babies stool after each feeding, while others stool daily or every 2 to 4 days. Pasty, seedy, curdy, or runny (like pea soup or heavy cream) stools are all

General
Principles

Common
Symptoms

Emergencies
and Traumas

Minor
Infections

Infectious
Diseases

Parenting
Concerns

normal. Normal stool color is mustard yellow, but it may also be green or brown. Breast-fed babies usually have looser and more frequent stools than formula-fed babies. *Straining* while stooling is common and does not indicate a problem. If the stools become hard like pebbles, or watery with only small flecks of solid, they are not normal. When such stools occur three or four times in a row, intervention may be necessary.

■ Care of the Diaper Area and Skin

When changing diapers, urine and stool should be washed from the baby's bottom with plain water. A bland soap may occasionally be necessary. Packaged *moist* wipes are useful, but those that contain alcohol may burn or irritate the baby's skin. *Petroleum jelly* applied to the diaper area is an inexpensive way to protect skin from the adverse effects of contact with urine and stool.

Mild *diaper rash* is best treated with a bland protective ointment containing zinc oxide. These *ointments* can be removed easily by gently wiping them off with baby oil. Successful treatment of diaper rash requires exposing the affected area to the air. Cutting out the elastic leg bands is a useful alternative when the baby cannot be left with the diaper area exposed. If the rash becomes worse despite treatment, especially when it looks like a weeping burn or pus-filled pimples, the skin may be infected, and evaluation and intervention may be indicated.

If a baby boy has been circumcised, no special care of the *circumcision* is necessary. To protect the skin from urine and stool, petroleum jelly may be applied with each diaper change for the first week or so until healing is complete. An *uncircumcised* penis also requires no special care. The foreskin should not be retracted forcefully, as irritation or bleeding may result. Cleaning beneath a tight foreskin is not necessary for good hygiene during infancy.

Female babies sometimes have a thick creamy or bloody *vaginal discharge,* caused by placental transfer of maternal hormones. It is normal and should be no cause for concern. When discharge occurs, the baby's vaginal labial folds should be cleansed gently from front to back (top to bottom) with water or baby oil.

Dry skin can be treated with a bland baby lotion. If a heat rash develops, *baby powder* with a corn starch base may be applied. The baby's skin should not be powdered directly because he or she may breathe in the powder. Instead, powder should be sprinkled into a hand and then wiped onto the baby.

Many babies develop mild *jaundice* or yellowing of the skin that is harmless. It may require treatment if it reaches very high levels, if it is associated with blood group incompatibility, or if the infant is premature or ill. Skin described as having a "pumpkin" color or if jaundice is visible on the baby's palms, soles, or stomach, further evaluation is needed. When looking for jaundice, parents should be instructed to examine the baby in daylight or under fluorescent light, and the baby should not be wearing yellow garments.

■ Care of the Umbilicus

The base of the umbilicus (belly button) should be swabbed with alcohol once or twice a day to dry the area and prevent infection. Air-drying should be used when practical. The umbilical scab will usually fall off 5 days to 4 weeks after birth. Associated *bleeding* or *oozing* requires no treatment other than swabbing the area clean. A foul odor or a spreading area of redness around or above the umbilicus suggests the possibility of infection and should be evaluated further.

■ Bathing

Sponge baths may be given daily or every 2 days until the baby's belly button is healed and dry; parents may then place the baby in a tub. Use of a bland soap that is rinsed completely from the skin helps to prevent irritation and rashes.

■ Visitors

During the first 2 to 4 weeks, the number of people who handle the baby should be limited to close friends and relatives. Those who have colds should avoid contact with the baby whenever possible. If the person handling the baby has a cold or other illness, strict *hand washing* is necessary. *Cigarette smoke* is not good for the parents or the baby and should be avoided, especially in areas where the baby sleeps or plays.

■ Taking the Baby Out

In emergency situations, the baby may be taken out at any time if dressed properly to prevent chilling. Depending on weather conditions, *planned walks* may be started when the baby is a few weeks old. Places that are heavily crowded should be avoided when practical. Beginning with the baby's trip home from the hospital, infants traveling in a car should *always* be strapped into an approved *car seat.*

■ Sleeping Positions

Babies should sleep on a firm crib mattress or a similar *firm surface.* Waterbeds, quilts, comforters, sheepskin, or other soft surfaces are *not* safe for the baby. During the first 5 or 6 months, the *safest sleeping position* appears to be on the side or back. There is evidence to suggest that the stomach-down (prone) sleeping position may increase the incidence of sudden infant death syndrome (SIDS).

■ Pacifiers

The sucking reflex in the newborn period can be strong, and allowing an infant to use a pacifier may help during fussy episodes.

■ Postpartum "Blues"

After giving birth, some mothers experience crying spells and feelings of depression in the hospital or shortly after taking the baby home. These may occur because of hormonal changes following delivery, nervousness about starting the new job of being a mother, uncertainty about which or

General
Principles

Common
Symptoms

Emergencies
and Traumas

Minor
Infections

Infectious
Diseases

Parenting
Concerns

Infant
Care

whose advice to accept, and general fatigue. They are common and normal and will usually disappear after a few weeks. Sleep deprivation may masquerade as depression causing an inability to concentrate, lack of desire to maintain social contacts, loss of appetite, and a lack of self-worth. If these feelings persist for longer than one month, and they are not the result of an obvious cause, counseling should be considered.

■ The First Doctor Visit

The first baby visit is usually scheduled 2 to 4 weeks after the baby's discharge from the hospital. It may be scheduled sooner if there is a specific medical problem. Parents should be instructed to make a list of their concerns before this first "well-baby" check-up. To avoid distractions at this important visit, it is best if parents can leave other children at home or make arrangements for them to be supervised.

Notes

General Principles

Common Symptoms

Emergencies and Traumas

Minor Infections

Infectious Diseases

Parenting Concerns

Infant Care

General
Principles

Common
Symptoms

Emergencies
and Traumas

Minor
Infections

Infectious
Diseases

Parenting
Concerns

Infant
Care

Notes

_____

_____

_____

_____

_____

_____

_____

_____

_____

_____

_____

_____

_____

_____

_____

_____

_____

_____

_____

_____

_____

_____

_____

General
Principles

Common
Symptoms

Emergencies
and Traumas

Minor
Infections

Appendix I

The Receptionist's Manual

Triage Instructions

Calls Requiring Immediate Attention

- Severe trauma, pain, or parental anxiety
- Calls from a physician or hospital about an ill patient

SCREENING QUESTION. "The doctor is with a patient. Would you like me to interrupt her for you?"

- Calls the parent believes are an emergency

SCREENING QUESTION. "Is this problem an emergency?"

Calls Requiring Attention in the Near Future

- Acute illness (fever, upper respiratory tract infection, cough, vomiting, etc.)
- Calls from pharmacies concerning prescriptions
- Minor trauma

Routine (Nonemergent) Calls

- Infant care (feeding, bathing, diaper rash, etc.)
- Behavioral and school problems
- Prescription refills
- Hospital or office business (billing, schedules, etc.)

Infectious
Diseases

Parenting
Concerns

Infant
Care

Jeffrey L. Brown: *Pediatric Telephone Medicine: Principles, Triage, and Advice,*
Second Edition. Copyright © 1994 J. B. Lippincott Company

General
Principles

Common
Symptoms

Emergencies
and Traumas

Minor
Infections

Infectious
Diseases

Parenting
Concerns

Infant
Care

Dietary Advice

Clear Liquids To Be Used for Vomiting

- Fruit juice diluted with water
- Soda with gas stirred out (*not* diet soda)
- Broth
- Weak tea with sugar
- Gelatin desert in liquid form (no artificial sweeteners)

Bland Diet To Be Used for Diarrhea

- Boiled egg, potato, chicken, beef.
- Cereals with lactose-reduced milk.
- Pasta with bland sauce.
- Rice, bread, toast, or crackers.
- Vegetables; limited amounts of fruits that are not packed in sugar syrups.
- Beverages: lactose-reduced milk, soy formula, commercial electrolyte solutions, water (if taken with other solids).
  Avoid foods and beverages with high sugar content. These include soda (high in fructose), fruit juices, ice cream, and gelatin deserts. Consider giving them in diluted form in small amounts.

Note
- Red-colored liquids can sometimes be confused with blood. Preferred clear juices include apple and white grape juice. Clear sodas include ginger ale and lemon-flavored drinks.
- Clear liquids should contain calories. Avoid use of diet sodas and plain water.

Milk and Milk-product-Free Diet

Avoid any foods labeled as containing milk, cheese, cream, ice cream, yogurt, whey, or milk solids.

   Beware of restaurant foods that may contain milk or cheese. These include baked goods, bread crumbs, and breaded foods; sausage meats including hot dogs; sauces (including tomato sauce) and gravy; sherbert; chocolate.

Acceptable foods usually include

- Any food labeled "Kosher-Parve."
- Breads: Rye, italian, French, hard rolls, pumpernickel, bagels.
- Spreads: Mayonnaise, nondairy margarine, jam, and jelly.
- Deserts: Ices, sorbet, tofu, *e.g.,* "Tofuti," and many fruit pops.

General Principles

Common Symptoms

Emergencies and Traumas

Minor Infections

Infectious Diseases

Parenting Concerns

Infant Care

Telephone Numbers

Professional and Ancillary Staff Members

Name/Address: _____ **Phone:** ____ _____

_____ ____ _____

_____ ____ _____

_____ **Fax:** ____ _____

Name/Address: _____ **Phone:** ____ _____

_____ ____ _____

_____ ____ _____

_____ **Fax:** ____ _____

Name/Address: _____ **Phone:** ____ _____

_____ ____ _____

_____ ____ _____

_____ **Fax:** ____ _____

Name/Address: _____ **Phone:** ____ _____

_____ ____ _____

_____ ____ _____

_____ **Fax:** ____ _____

Name/Address: _____ **Phone:** ____ _____

_____ ____ _____

_____ ____ _____

_____ **Fax:** ____ _____

Name/Address: _____ **Phone:** ____ _____

_____ ____ _____

_____ ____ _____

_____ **Fax:** ____ _____

Pharmacies, Consultants, Suppliers, Insurance Companies

Name/Address: _____ Phone: ____ _____
_____ ____ _____
_____ ____ _____
_____ Fax: ____ _____

Name/Address: _____ Phone: ____ _____
_____ ____ _____
_____ ____ _____
_____ Fax: ____ _____

Name/Address: _____ Phone: ____ _____
_____ ____ _____
_____ ____ _____
_____ Fax: ____ _____

Name/Address: _____ Phone: ____ _____
_____ ____ _____
_____ ____ _____
_____ Fax: ____ _____

Name/Address: _____ Phone: ____ _____
_____ ____ _____
_____ ____ _____
_____ Fax: ____ _____

Name/Address: _____ Phone: ____ _____
_____ ____ _____
_____ ____ _____
_____ Fax: ____ _____

Name/Address: _____ Phone: ____ _____
_____ ____ _____
_____ ____ _____
_____ Fax: ____ _____

General Principles

Common Symptoms

Emergencies and Traumas

Minor Infections

Infectious Diseases

Parenting Concerns

Infant Care

Name/Address: _____   **Phone:** ____ _____

_____   ____ _____

_____   ____ _____

_____   **Fax:** ____ _____

Name/Address: _____   **Phone:** ____ _____

_____   ____ _____

_____   ____ _____

_____   **Fax:** ____ _____

Name/Address: _____   **Phone:** ____ _____

_____   ____ _____

_____   ____ _____

_____   **Fax:** ____ _____

Name/Address: _____   **Phone:** ____ _____

_____   ____ _____

_____   ____ _____

_____   **Fax:** ____ _____

Name/Address: _____   **Phone:** ____ _____

_____   ____ _____

_____   ____ _____

_____   **Fax:** ____ _____

Name/Address: _____   **Phone:** ____ _____

_____   ____ _____

_____   ____ _____

_____   **Fax:** ____ _____

278

General
Principles

Common
Symptoms

Emergencies
and Traumas

Minor
Infections

Infectious
Diseases

Parenting
Concerns

Infant
Care

Schedules for Physical Examinations and Immunizations

Physical Examinations

Examinations required at ages: _____ _____ _____ _____

_____ _____ _____ _____ _____ _____ _____ _____

Immunizations

Immunization: _____

Required at ages: _____ _____ _____ _____ _____ _____

Immunization: _____

Required at ages: _____ _____ _____ _____ _____ _____

Immunization: _____

Required at ages: _____ _____ _____ _____ _____ _____

Immunization: _____

Required at ages: _____ _____ _____ _____ _____ _____

Immunization: _____

Required at ages: _____ _____ _____ _____ _____ _____

Immunization: _____

Required at ages: _____ _____ _____ _____ _____ _____

Immunization: _____

Required at ages: _____ _____ _____ _____ _____ _____

General Principles

Immunization: _____

Required at ages: _____ _____ _____ _____ _____ _____

Common Symptoms

Immunization: _____

Required at ages: _____ _____ _____ _____ _____ _____

Immunization: _____

Required at ages: _____ _____ _____ _____ _____ _____

Emergencies and Traumas

Immunization: _____

Required at ages: _____ _____ _____ _____ _____ _____

Immunization: _____

Required at ages: _____ _____ _____ _____ _____ _____

Minor Infections

Immunization: _____

Required at ages: _____ _____ _____ _____ _____ _____

Immunization: _____

Required at ages: _____ _____ _____ _____ _____ _____

Infectious Diseases

Immunization: _____

Required at ages: _____ _____ _____ _____ _____ _____

Immunization: _____

Required at ages: _____ _____ _____ _____ _____ _____

Parenting Concerns

Immunization: _____

Required at ages: _____ _____ _____ _____ _____ _____

Immunization: _____

Required at ages: _____ _____ _____ _____ _____ _____

Infant Care

280

Commonly Used
OTC Medications

Medication: _____

    Age/weight: _____ _____ _____ _____ _____

       Dosage: _____ _____ _____ _____ _____

Medication: _____

    Age/weight: _____ _____ _____ _____ _____

       Dosage: _____ _____ _____ _____ _____

Medication: _____

    Age/weight: _____ _____ _____ _____ _____

       Dosage: _____ _____ _____ _____ _____

Medication: _____

    Age/weight: _____ _____ _____ _____ _____

       Dosage: _____ _____ _____ _____ _____

Medication: _____

    Age/weight: _____ _____ _____ _____ _____

       Dosage: _____ _____ _____ _____ _____

Medication: _____

    Age/weight: _____ _____ _____ _____ _____

       Dosage: _____ _____ _____ _____ _____

Jeffrey L. Brown: *Pediatric Telephone Medicine: Principles, Triage, and Advice,*
Second Edition. Copyright © 1994 J. B. Lippincott Company

Medication: _____

     Age/weight: _____ _____ _____ _____ _____

     Dosage: _____ _____ _____ _____ _____

Medication: _____

     Age/weight: _____ _____ _____ _____ _____

     Dosage: _____ _____ _____ _____ _____

Medication: _____

     Age/weight: _____ _____ _____ _____ _____

     Dosage: _____ _____ _____ _____ _____

Medication: _____

     Age/weight: _____ _____ _____ _____ _____

     Dosage: _____ _____ _____ _____ _____

Medication: _____

     Age/weight: _____ _____ _____ _____ _____

     Dosage: _____ _____ _____ _____ _____

Medication: _____

     Age/weight: _____ _____ _____ _____ _____

     Dosage: _____ _____ _____ _____ _____

Medication: _____

     Age/weight: _____ _____ _____ _____ _____

     Dosage: _____ _____ _____ _____ _____

282

Travel Instructions to the Office

(Use a format that can be faxed when necessary.)

_____

_____

_____

_____

_____

_____

_____

_____

_____

_____

_____

_____

_____

_____

_____

_____

_____

_____

_____

_____

_____

_____

_____

_____

General Principles

Common Symptoms

Emergencies and Traumas

Minor Infections

Infectious Diseases

Parenting Concerns

Infant Care

Billing, Insurance, and Other Office Business Policies

Common Symptoms

Emergencies and Traumas

Minor Infections

Infectious Diseases

Parenting Concerns

Infant Care

Jeffrey L. Brown: *Pediatric Telephone Medicine: Principles, Triage, and Advice,* Second Edition. Copyright © 1994 J. B. Lippincott Company

Patient Instructions

The following is a list of instructions that might be included in a patient information booklet for distribution at the practice setting. You might wish to copy it in its entirety, to use only the general rules for calling, to add specific office policy, or to modify the screening questions.

When and How To Call Your Child's Doctor

General Rules For Calling The Doctor Or Nurse

- When calling for *nonurgent matters* such as well-baby advice, prescription refills, billing matters, or appointments, call during office hours whenever possible. Ask the receptionist for the best hours to call.
- When calling for an *emergency* tell the office receptionist or answering service operator that "this call is an emergency" so that you can be put in touch with the doctor as quickly as possible.
- After calling for any problem, ask when the doctor or nurse is *most likely to return your call.*
- If you do not receive a *return call* within a reasonable period of time, always call our office back to be certain a misunderstanding has not taken place.
- Have paper and pencil ready to *write down instructions* you may receive. Also, have your *pharmacy's telephone number* handy.
- *Give the following information* at every call: your child's name, age, and sex, the telephone number(s) and time(s) when you can be reached, and your child's most important symptom (such as earache).
- Give the *most important information* first and try to be brief when giving symptoms to the receptionist or answering service operator. For example, "My child has had a fever and vomiting for two days."
- A *parent's intuition* is very important. If you feel very nervous about your child's condition, say so. If you believe that your child looks well despite his or her present symptoms, report that also.
- *Report any chronic illnesses* your child has, such as diabetes or asthma, any *immunizations* (shots) your child has received re-

Emergencies
and Traumas

Minor
Infections

Infectious
Diseases

Parenting
Concerns

Infant
Care

General Principles

Common Symptoms

Emergencies and Traumas

Minor Infections

Infectious Diseases

Parenting Concerns

Infant Care

cently, and any medicines or other *treatments* your child is presently receiving.

- If medicines are prescribed, *report any allergies* that your child is known to have.
- Before calling, be aware of which *children's medicines are available* in your home.
- If an examination is not necessary, at the *completion of your call* you should know the most likely cause of your child's condition, which medicines or treatments should be given, and what signs or symptoms to watch for. You should also know under what circumstances you should call the doctor or nurse back.
- If you don't *understand the instructions* given by the doctor or nurse, ask to have them repeated.
- If you are instructed to come to the doctor's office or to go to the emergency room, obtain *travel instructions* before leaving home. When traveling in a car, even during an emergency, drive slowly and carefully, and use a restraining car seat for your child. If you feel too nervous to drive, call a friend or a taxi. If an ambulance is needed, the doctor or nurse may be able to call it for you.

When To Call Immediately for an Infant Younger than 3 Months Old

- If the baby is lethargic (very sleepy or difficult to arouse), has poor color, or appears limp and unresponsive.
- If the baby has a rectal temperature of 101°F or higher.
- If the baby refuses to eat three or four times in a row.
- If the child's hands or feet have a yellow "jaundiced" color or if the baby develops pumpkin-colored skin.
- If the baby has repeated bouts of diarrhea or vomiting.
- If the baby has a labored, wheezing, or "grunting" breathing pattern that lasts longer than one-half hour.
- If your child has an illness associated with a rash that looks like bleeding under the skin.
- If you feel very nervous about your baby's illness or general condition.

When To Call Immediately for an Older Child

- If your child seems unresponsive, does not make eye contact with you, or has cold and clammy skin that is not associated with vomiting.
- If your child looks much sicker than usual with a "routine" illness.
- If your child has an illness associated with a rash that looks like bleeding under the skin.
- If your child has any symptom that you believe to be unusual or

286

frightening. This might include labored breathing, severe headache, or very high fever.

When To Call Immediately after Trauma or Injury

- If your child has struck his or her head and has lost consciousness, has nausea or vomiting, or complains of severe headache. Also report any of the following: mental confusion, unbalanced walking, poor coordination, loss of memory, or a discharge coming from one or both ears.
- If there is a persistent swelling, tenderness, or deformity of the injured part.
- If your child refuses to use an injured extremity for more than one-half hour.
- If there is a deep puncture wound; a cut longer than $\frac{1}{2}$ inch; or your child has not received a tetanus shot within the past 5 to 10 years.
- If there is injury to an eye that causes redness, pain, or tearing for more than 15 minutes.
- If your child has been bitten by an animal, and the bite has gone through the skin.
- If you need first-aid instructions for uncontrolled bleeding or other problems.
- If you believe that your child may have swallowed a toxic or poisonous substance.

When To Call for a Symptom

- If you are concerned about the child's general appearance.
- If the symptom seems to be getting progressively worse or lasts longer than expected.
- If fever of more than 101°F has persisted for longer than 24 hours.
- If cough, cold, sore throat, or runny nose has lasted longer than 48 hours.
- If vomiting has lasted longer than 8 hours or diarrhea longer than 24 hours. Or when there is blood in the stool or vomit.
- If the child has severe stomach pains lasting longer than 4 hours.
- If the symptom seems more severe than it has in the past.
- If your child has a rash or other problem and you are not sure what is causing it.
- If you are not certain whether the child needs to be seen by the doctor or nurse.

Emergencies
and Traumas

Minor
Infections

Infectious
Diseases

Parenting
Concerns

Infant
Care

General
Principles

Common
Symptoms

Emergencies
and Traumas

Minor
Infections

Infectious
Diseases

Parenting
Concerns

Infant
Care

References

Preface, Introduction, Basic Elements of the Telephone Call

American Academy of Pediatrics, Committee on Practice and Ambulatory Medicine. *Management of pediatric practice.* Elk Grove Village, IL: American Academy of Pediatrics, 1986. Pp. 28–36.

American Academy of Pediatrics, Committee on Standards of Child Health Care. *Standards of child health care,* 2nd ed. Evanston IL: American Academy of Pediatrics, 1972.

Barton EL, Brown JL, Curtis P, et al. Making phone care good care. *Patient Care* 1992; 103–118.

Bergman AB, Dassel SW, Wedgwood RJ. Time motion study of practicing pediatricians. *Pediatrics* 1966; 38:254–263.

Brown JL. The telephone in pediatric practice. *Clin Pediatr* 1983; 22:777.

Brown JL. Telephone tyranny: How to overcome it. *Pediatr Mgmnt* 1992; Jun:15–28.

Brown JL. Telephone patient management. *Pediatr Basics* 1984; No. 9.

Brown JL. The telephone in pediatric practice. *Clin Pediatr* 1983; 22:777.

Brown JL. *The complete parents' guide to telephone medicine: When to call, what to ask, how to help,* 2nd ed. New York: Perigee; Putnam Publishing Group, 1988.

Brown JL. *Telephone medicine: A practical guide to pediatric telephone advice.* St. Louis: C.V. Mosby, 1980.

Brown SB, Eberle BJ. Use of the telephone by pediatric housestaff: A technique of pediatric care not taught. *J Pediatr* 1974; 84:117–119.

Caplan SE, Orr JT, Skulstad JR, Charney E. After hours telephone use in urban pediatric primary care centers. *Am J Dis Child* 1983; 137:879–882.

Caplan SE, Straus JH. Strategies for reducing inappropriate telephone calls. *Clin Pediatr* 1988; 27:236–239.

Curry TA, Schwartz MW. Telephone assessment of illness: What is being taught and learned? *Pediatrics* 1978; 62:603–605.

Curtis R. The telephone in medical practice. *J Fam Pract* 1978; 6:897–898.

Fosarelli P, Katz H. Residents on the phone. *Pediatrics* 1987; 79: 311–312.

Fosarelli PD. The telephone in pediatric medicine: A review. *Clin Pediatr* 1983; 22:293–296.

Fosarelli PD. The emphasis of telephone medicine in pediatric training programs. *Am J Dis Child* 1985; 139:555–557.

Fosarelli P, Schmitt B. Telephone dissatisfaction in pediatric practice: Denver and Baltimore. *Pediatrics* 1987; 80:28–31.

Goodman HC, Perrin EC. Evening telephone call management by nurse practitioners and physicians. *Nurs Res* 1979; 27:233–237.

Gorrell RL. Taming the terrible telephone. *Phys Mgmt* 1978; 18:40–42.

Greitzer L, Stapleton FB, Wright L, et al. Telephone assessment of illness by practicing pediatricians. *J Pediatr* 1976; 88:880–882.

Heagarty MC. The use of the telephone in pediatric practice. *In* Green M, ed. *Ambulatory pediatrics.* Philadelphia: W.B. Saunders, 1968. Pp. 136–138.

Heagarty MC. From house calls to telephone calls. *Am J Publ Health* 1978; 68:14–15.

Heagarty MC. The telephone syndrome. *Pediatrics* 1979; 64:696–697.

Holm RS: Good telephone technique aids in pediatric emergencies. *Mich Med* 1979; 78:124.

Katz HP, Pozen J, Mushlin AI. Quality assessment of a telephone care system utilizing nonphysician personnel. *Am J Public Health* 1978; 68:31–38.

Katz HP. *Telephone medicine triage and training: a handbook for primary health care professionals.* Philadelphia: F.A. Davis, 1990.

Leebov W, Vergare M, Scott G. Telephone tact and tactics. *In Patient satisfaction: A guide to practice enhancement.* Oradell, NJ: Medical Economics Books, 1990. Pp. 121–143.

General Principles

Common Symptoms

Emergencies and Traumas

Minor Infections

Infectious Diseases

Parenting Concerns

Infant Care

Levy JC, Rosenkranz J, Lamb GA, et al. Development and field testing of protocols for the management of pediatric telephone calls: Protocols for pediatric telephone calls. *Pediatrics* 1979; 64:558–563.

Levy JC, Strasser PH, Lamb GA, et al. Survey of telephone encounters in three pediatric practice sites. *Public Health Res* 1980; 95:324–328.

Mapes RW, Lewis EW Jr, Covell DG, et al. Feasibility study of a pediatric telephone consultation service. *Pediatrics* 1972; 50:307–311.

Ott JE, Bellaire J, Machotka P, et al. Patient management by telephone by child health associates and pediatric health officers. *J Med Educ* 1974; 49:596–600.

Poole SR, Schmitt BD, Carruth T, et al. After-hours telephone coverage: The application of an area-wide telephone triage and advice system for pediatric practices. *Pediatrics* 1993; 92:670.

Perrin EC, Goodman HC. Telephone management of acute pediatric illnesses. *N Engl J Med* 1978; 298:130–135.

Reece RM, Robertson LS, Alpert JJ. The telephone answering service: A survey of use by general practitioners and pediatricians in Massachusetts. *Clin Pediatr* 1972; 11:40–43.

Rosenkrans J, et al. *Pediatric telephone protocols.* Darien, CT: Patient Care Publications, 1979.

Schmitt BD. *Pediatric telephone advice: Guidelines for the health care provider on telephone triage and office management of common childhood syndromes.* Boston: Little, Brown, & Company, 1980.

Selbst SM, Korin J. The telephone in pediatric emergency medicine. *Pediatr Emerg Care* 1985; 1:108–110.

Smith SR, Fischer PM. Patient management by telephone: A training exercise for medical students. *J Fam Pract* 1980; 10:463–466.

Strain JE, Miller JD. The preparation, utilization, and evaluation of a registered nurse trained to give telephone advice in a private pediatric office. *Pediatrics* 1971; 47:1051–1055.

Strasser PH, Levy JC, Lamb GA, et al. Controlled clinical trial of telephone protocols. *Pediatrics* 1979; 64:553–557.

Thayer MB: Telephone management. *Pediatr Nurs* 1984; 10:121–154.

Tripp SL: What to ask and what to do when parents call about children's illnesses. *Nursing* 1974; 4:73–79.

General Principles

Common Symptoms

Emergencies and Traumas

Minor Infections

Infectious Diseases

Parenting Concerns

Infant Care

Tripp SL. Telephone techniques in pediatric practice. *Am J Nurs* 1971; 71:1722–1724.

Villarreal SF, Berman S, Groothuis JR, et al. Telephone encounters in a university pediatric group practice: A 2 year analysis of after-hours calls. *Clin Pediatr* 1984; 23:456–458.

Wood PR. Pediatric resident training in telephone management: A survey of training programs in the United States. *Pediatrics* 1986; 77: 822–825.

Wood PR, Littlefield JH, Foulds DM. Telephone management curriculum for pediatric interns: A controlled trial. *Pediatrics* 1992; 83:925.

Yankowski SZ, Yankowski JA, Malley JD, et al. Telephone triage by primary care physicians. *Pediatrics* 1992; 89:701.

Isaacman DJ, Verdile VP, Kohen FP. Pediatric telephone advice in the emergency department: Results of a mock scenario. *Pediatrics* 1992; 89:35.

Improving Communication Skills

American Medical Association, Department of Practice Management. *Winning ways with patients.* Chicago: American Medical Association, 1979.

American Medical Association, Department of Practice Management. *Talking with patients.* Chicago: American Medical Association, 1984.

Cassell EJ. *Talking with patients,* Vol. 1. Cambridge, MA: MIT Press, 1985.

Cahill M, ed. *Patient teaching.* Springhouse, PA: Nursing 89 Books, 1987.

Cline RJ. Interpersonal communication skills for enhancing physician–patient relationships. *Maryland State Med* 1983; 32(4):272–278.

Davis CM. *Patient practitioner interaction; an experimental manual for developing the art of health care.* Thorofare, NJ: Slack, 1989.

Frank MO. *How to get your point across in 30 seconds or less.* New York: Pocket Books, 1986.

Girard J. *How to sell yourself.* New York: Warner Books, 1979.

Gold SR. Patient communication begins with listening. *Amb Care* 1986; 6(5):36–37.

General Principles

Common Symptoms

Emergencies and Traumas

Minor Infections

Infectious Diseases

Parenting Concerns

Infant Care

General
Principles

Common
Symptoms

Emergencies
and Traumas

Minor
Infections

Infectious
Diseases

Parenting
Concerns

Infant
Care

Henderson G. The importance of physician-patient communication. *Hosp Phys* 1984; 20(7):32–33, 36.

Korsch BM, Negrete VF. Doctor–patient communication. *Sci Am* 1972; 227:66.

Korsch BM, Aley EF. Pediatric interviewing techniques. *In Current problems in pediatrics,* Vol. 3. Chicago: Year Book Medical Publishers, 1973.

Leebov W. *Service excellence: The customer relations strategy for health care.* American Hospital Publishing, 1988.

Leebov W, Vergare M, Scott G. *Patient satisfaction: A guide to practice enhancement.* Oradell, NJ: Medical Economics Books, 1990.

Ley P. *Communicating with patients: Improving communication, satisfaction and compliance.* New York: Croom Helm, 1988.

MacHaffie RA. Make your patients feel you really understand them. *Physician's Management* 1982; 22(11):151–153, 156, 158.

O'Donnell WE. Assumptions that can ruin patient relations. *Medical Economics* 1988; 65(24):135–136, 138.

Posner RB. Physician–patient communication. *Am J Med* 1984; 77(3A): 59–64.

Roberts JR. Physician–patient relationships. *Amb Care* 1986; 6:45.

Scroggins LW. Let patients know how good you are. *Medical Economics* 1988; 65(6):173–174, 176.

Waitzkin H. Doctor–patient communication. *JAMA* 1984: 252(7): 2441–2446.

Telephone Record Keeping and Liability

American Academy of Pediatrics, Committee on Practice and Ambulatory Medicine. The office telephone: Triage, training and technique. *In Management of pediatric practice,* 2nd ed. Elk Grove Village, IL: American Academy of Pediatrics, 1991. P. 38.

Brown JL. *Pediatric telephone medicine: Principles, triage, and advice.* Philadelphia: J.B. Lippincott, 1991. P. 18.

Cohn B. Office malpractice pitfalls. *Pediatr Ann* 1991; 20:69.

Fulginiti VA. The big 8: Major malpractice traps in pediatrics. *Pediatr Mgmnt* 1993; Apr:40.

Katz HP, Wick W. Malpractice, meningitis, and the telephone. *Pediatr Ann* 1991; 20:85.

Katz HP. *Telephone medicine, triage and training: A handbook for professionals.* Philadelphia: F.A. Davis, 1990.

Medical–Legal Issues in Pediatrics, 18th ed. Columbus, OH: Ross Roundtable; Aug 1987. P. 2.

Ricci JA, Lambert RL, Steffes DG. Pediatrics and professional liability. *Pediatr Emerg Care* 1986; 2:106.

Richards EP, Rathbun KC. *Law and the physician: A practical guide.* Boston: Little, Brown & Company, 1993. Pp. 115, 440.

Schmitt B. *Pediatric telephone advice.* Boston: Little, Brown & Company, 1980.

Vogt LB, Armitage DT. Physician patient relationship. *In* American College of Legal Medicine. *Legal Medicine: Legal dynamics of medical encounters.* St. Louis: C.V. Mosby, Co. 1988. P. 188.

Patient Relations: The Irate Patient

Alexander P, Salmon P. How to manage patient complaints. *Physician's Management* 1984; 24(10):294–295, 298–301, 305.

Allaire B, McNeill R. *Teaching patient relations in hospitals: The hows and the whys.* Chicago: American Hospital Publishing, 1984.

Alper PR. Surefire steps to soothe the savage patient. *Medical Economics* 1985; 62(6):131–132, 135–136.

Comeau JF. How to manage patient complaints. *Physician's Management* 1988; 28(4):148–149, 152–155.

Ehrlich A. Handling the irate caller. *Dental Economics* 1984; 74(7): 59–60.

Garbelt A. Helping patients you don't like. *Physician's Management* 1983; 23(3):289–291.

Hellstern RA. Managing patient complaints. *Amb Care* 1986; 6(3):10–11.

Kazemek EA, Peterson KE. Improving complaint management skills. *Healthcare Financial Management* 1987; 41(10):122–123.

Lewis B. Effective ways of managing the difficult patient. *Physician's Management* 1986; 26(3):104–105, 108–109, 112, 117–118, 120.

General Principles

Common Symptoms

Emergencies and Traumas

Minor Infections

Infectious Diseases

Parenting Concerns

Infant Care

Oppenheim G. How to diffuse a hostile patient. *Medical Economics* 1988; 65(17):125–126, 128, 130, 133–134.

Common Symptomatic Complaints, Trauma and Other Emergency Problems, Infectious Diseases, Common Parenting Concerns, Care of Newborn Infants

American Academy of Pediatrics, Committee on Infectious Diseases. *Report of the Committee on Infectious Diseases.* Elk Grove Village, IL: American Academy of Pediatrics, 1991.

American Medical Association. *Children: How to understand their symptoms.* New York: Random House, 1986.

Barkin RM, Rosen P. *Emergency pediatrics: A guide to ambulatory care,* 4th ed. St. Louis: C.V. Mosby, 1994.

Burg FD, Ingelfinger JR, Wald ER. *Gellis and Kagen's current pediatric therapy,* 14th ed. Philadelphia: W.B. Saunders, 1993.

Crain EF, Gershel JC, Gallagher EJ. *Clinical manual of emergency pediatrics,* 2nd ed. New York: McGraw Hill, 1992.

Johnson KK, ed. *The Harriet Lane handbook: A manual for pediatric house officers.* St. Louis: C.V. Mosby, 1993.

Oski FA, DeAngelis CD, Feigin RD, Warshaw SB. *Principles and practice of pediatrics.* Philadelphia: J.B. Lippincott, 1990.

Plaut TF. *Children with asthma: A manual for parents,* 2nd ed. Amherst: Pedipress, Inc., 1984.

Schulman ST, MacKendrick WP, Stamos JK. *Handbook of pediatric infectious disease and antimicrobial therapy.* St. Louis: Mosby Year Book, 1993.

Stockman JA, Corden TE, Kin JJ. *The pediatric book of lists: A primer of differential diagnosis in pediatrics.* St. Louis: Mosby Year Book, 1991.

Index

Exposure to infectious diseases,
233–236
Eye
infection of, 185–186, 205
irrigation of, 145–146
strain of, 117
trauma to, 145–146

F
Falls, 139–140
Fearfulness, 254
Feeding(s)
breast, 263–264
calculation of, 104
formula, 265–266
impaired, 244, 252–253, 263
schedule for, 266
Fever, 53–54
convulsions with, 57–58
discussion of, 55–58
in infants, 263
intermittent, 83
phobia about, 55–56
rash with, 57
from roseola, 227
stiff neck with, 57
treatment for, 54–55
Fever blisters, 181
Fifth disease, 207–208
Fissure, anal, 103
Fluoride, 266
Follow-up
to office visit, 34–35
of telephone call, 13, 44
Food, solid, 266
Foreign body ingestion, 165–166
Formula feeding, 265–266
Fructose intolerance, 94
Funerals, 255
Fungal infections, 125

G
Gastroenteritis, 93, 103, 113
Gastroesophageal reflux, 103

Gastrointestinal symptoms,
91–113
Genital irritation, 120
German measles, 209–210
exposure to, 233

H
Haemophilus influenzae, 79, 126,
234–235
Head lice, 183–184
exposure to, 234
Head trauma, 141–142
Headache, 115–117
Heat rash, 127–128
Hematuria, 121
Hemorrhage, 135
Hemorrhagic rash, 126
Henoch-Schönlein purpura, 94,
126
Hepatitis, 211–212
exposure to, 234
Hernia, 103
Herpangina, 9
Herpes simplex infection, 181
Herpes virus 6, 227, 228
Herpes zoster, 205
Hidden agenda, 12–13
HIV. *See* Human immunodefi-
ciency virus (HIV).
Hives, 126
treatment for, 124
Hold button, 5–6, 36
Hospitalization, 34
Human bites, 155–156
Human immunodeficiency virus
(HIV), 203, 233
Hyperactive airway disease, 85–89

I
Ibuprofen, 55
Ice packs
for athletic injury, 138
for bites, 151, 153, 155
for trauma, 135, 143, 145

Triage (*continued*)
principles of, 6–7
by receptionist, 38–39, 273

U
Umbilicus, care of, 268
Upper respiratory infection (URI),
67, 81–84
nose bleed from, 158
treatment of, 82
Urination, 251–252
obstructed, 94
pain on, 119–121
Urine specimen, 121
Urticaria, 126
treatment for, 124
Uveitis, 186

V
Vaginal discharge, 195–197, 267
Vaporizer, 9
for cough, 66
for croup, 70
for nose bleeds, 158
for respiratory infection, 82–84
Varicella, 126, 203–205
exposure to, 233
Vascular headaches, 117
Viral disease. *See specific types,*
e.g., Fifth disease.

Visitors, of infants, 268
Vitamins, 253
in formula, 266
for infants, 265
toxicity of, 169
Voice-mail systems, 37
Vomiting, 111–113
after poisoning, 168
diet after, 274
in infants, 263
treatment for, 112

W
Waiting period, 6–7
Well-baby check-up, 270, 279
Wellness-bias, 8, 9, 26
Wheezing, 85–90
etiology of, 88
prevention of, 89
treatment for, 86, 89
Whooping cough, 67, 231–232
exposure to, 236
Working, ambivalent feelings
about, 255–256

X
X-ray films
for foreign bodies, 165–166
for head trauma, 142
for nose trauma, 143–144